Health Through Public Policy

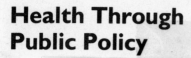

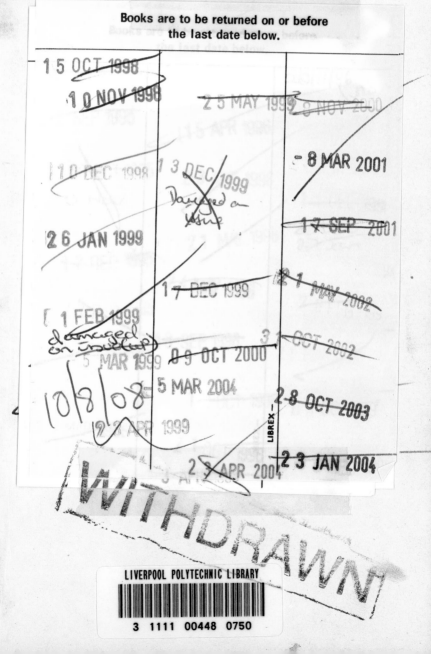

Health Through Public Policy

The greening
f public health

d by

er Draper

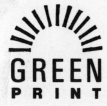

GREEN
PRINT

First published in 1991 by
Green Print
an imprint of The Merlin Press
10 Malden Road, London NW5 3HR

ISBN 1 85425 045 0

1 2 3 4 5 6 7 8 9 10 :: 99 98 97 96 95 94 93 92 91

Phototypeset by Computerset, Harmondsworth

Printed in England by Biddles Ltd., Guildford, Surrey on recycled paper

Contents

Contributors

Lee Adams was born and brought up in East London and began her working life as a teacher. Worked in NHS health education/promotion in London, Cambridge and Salford. Formerly the Director of Professional and Community Development at the Health Education Authority, she is currently the Director of Health Promotion for Sheffield Health Authority.

Peter Allen worked for local authorities in the South and the North before joining Oxford City Council in the mid-1970s. He is a founder member of the Institution of Environmental Health Officers' Health Promotion Committee, a member of the Health Education Authority's Environmental Health Advisory Committee and a part-time lecturer at Oxford University's School of Medicine and General Practice.

Victor Anderson is co-author with Michael Jacobs of *The Green Economy* (1991). Author of *Alternative Economic Indicators* (1990). Member, Projects Committee, New Economics Foundation.

John Clark. With Oxfam since 1979, mostly as Development Policy Advisor and Campaigns Manager, also responsible for representing Oxfam on the debt crisis, the World Bank's role and other development issues. Initiated in 1981 the Independent Group on British Aid which reports on government aid policy. His book *For Richer For Poorer* is on western connections with world hunger (Oxfam, 1986). Also author of *Zambia; Debt and Poverty* (Oxfam, 1989), *Democratizing Development* (Earthscan, 1991).

Peter Draper. Independent consultant in public health and emeritus consultant to Guy's Hospital where he previously planned (with Tony Smart) and then directed the Unit for the Study of Health Policy. A keen organic allotment gardener, he has been ecologically oriented since his sixth-form days. Founding member of the Public Health Alliance. Joint author of *Health, Money and the NHS* (1976), *Health, the Mass Media and the NHS* (1977), *Rethinking Community Medicine* (1979).

Phil Fryer. Health Liaison Officer, Oxford City Council, since 1984, has been developing a Healthy Cities Strategy for the City. Active as a commissioner of Oxford Health Authority's Public Health Commission.

Jenny Griffiths. General Manager of Oxfordshire Family Health Services Authority since 1989, with a previous career in health promotion, public health and health services planning in London, and with Oxford Regional Health Authority from 1985.

Trevor Hancock. Public health consultant who specialises in health promotion, healthy public policy and healthy cities in Canada and internationally. Has a long-standing commitment to the conserver or sustainable society, to ecological politics, and to the links between sustainability, equity and health.

Reg Harman worked for British Rail, a transport consultancy and the University of East Anglia in various posts involving economic and social planning of transport before joining Hertfordshire County Council's transport co-ordination unit. Currently senior planning officer developing the county's strategic policy and information.

Stanley Harrison, freelance editor and journalist, ex-GLC consultant, specialises in press history and economics. Author of *Poor Men's Guardians*.

Carol Haslam was first a social studies lecturer and trainee psychotherapist, then a producer in the BBC's Open University department, making programmes in social science and community health. She joined Channel 4 as Commissioning Editor for documentaries, including a weekly health slot. Now Managing Director of Hawkshead, an independent production company.

Mayer Hillman. Senior Fellow at the (London) Policy Studies Institute since 1970, researching policies on transport and road safety, energy use and conservation. He recently completed a study of the costs and benefits for the UK of putting the clock one hour ahead of its current setting throughout the year. He is presently involved in a study on a resource-conscious society.

David Keen is researching the politics of hunger at St. Antony's College, Oxford. He has worked as a consultant in the field of emergency relief and as a journalist with McGraw-Hill.

Jennifer Lisle. Occupational physician since 1975 with a background in public health. In 1985 founded Joint Research and Health Advisers, a consultancy in preventive and occupational medicine. Particular interests: mental health at work; management of organisational change and stress-related problems; counselling.

Ged Moran. Formerly Health Liaison Officer and subsequently Health Advisor to the London Borough of Greenwich, and then Health Liaison Officer in Leeds City Council's Health Unit. Now a consultant with the Health Policy Advisory Unit, a consultancy specialising in health policy and public health issues. Author of a number of articles on local authorities and health.

Jean Orr. Lecturer in nursing studies at Manchester University and an elected member of the English National Board for Nursing, Midwifery and Health Visiting. Research interests: women's health and community assessment.

Christopher Robbins is an independent food and health consultant working across all sectors of the food chain to develop national food and health policies. He is also a writer, broadcaster and trainer. After qualifying as an agricultural scientist in Australia he worked in Africa on rural development planning before spending seven years at the Centre for Agricultural Strategy, Reading University. Recent books include *The Healthy Catering Manual* (1989) and *Poisoned Harvest: The Consumer Guide to Pesticides* (1990).

Hilary Rose is Professor of Social Policy and Director of the West Yorkshire Centre for Research on Women. For some years she has worked with and written about social movements and their relationship to the formation of new health and welfare thinking and organisational forms. She has served as a social science consultant to the WHO European Region's Health Promotion division as part of the Healthy Cities initiative and in the development of Healthy Public Policy. And she hates writing short CVs almost more than any other writing task.

Eric B. Ross. American anthropologist; senior lecturer and director of the programme in human ecology, Huddersfield Polytechnic. Editor, *Beyond the Myths of Culture* (1980), co-editor, *Food and Evolution: Toward a Theory of Human Food Habits* (1987), co-author, *Death, Sex and Fertility: Population Regulation in Preindustrial and Developing Societies* (1987). In preparation: *English Feast, Irish Famine.*

Colin Thunhurst. Lecturer in quantitative methods for planning and management at Nuffield Institute for Health Service Studies, University of Leeds. Director of the Community Operational Research Unit at the Northern College of Residential Adult Education. Studied health inequalities in Sheffield and Stoke-on-Trent. Involved with the UK Healthy Cities Network and individual authorities pursuing Health For All programmes to develop core indicators. Author of *It Makes You Sick – The Politics of the NHS,* which includes proposals for democratising the NHS.

Jo Tunnard. Director of the Family Rights Group, which advises families with children in care, trains social workers and lawyers, and comments on central and local government policy relating to child care law and professional practice. Formerly Deputy Director, Child Poverty Action Group.

Steve Watkins is Director of Public Health, Stockport Health Authority; President of the Medical Practitioners' Union; Deputy Chairman, Annual

Conference of Community Medicine and Community Health. Author of *Medicine & Labour; the Politics of a Profession* and co-author of *Unemployment: Challenge and Public Health*. Has special interest in relationships between economic activity and health and is Convenor of the Unemployment and Health Study Group and Chairman of the Transport and Health Group.

Steve Webster has been involved in researching the arms business for a number of years. He has worked for the Campaign Against Arms Trade, the United Nations Association, the Ethical Investment Research Service (EIRIS) and New Consumer. He now works in the Information and Planning section of Leeds Social Services Department.

Patti White, former deputy director of Action on Smoking and Health (ASH) UK, is currently freelancing in health promotion after working with an international health organisation as a consultant on tobacco.

Foreword

The current controversies in the National Health Service can be read two ways: as the inevitable end-product of an implacably hostile government endeavouring to choke the life out of the NHS by drawing the purse strings tighter and tighter; or as the final confirmation of the inherent un-manageability of a service that probably couldn't cope however much money we chose to chuck at it.

In reality, it's probably a bit of both. There's no denying the hostility of the Thatcher governments for the doctors and ancillary workers within the NHS. And from a Green perspective, there's no denying the idiocy of trying to keep a nation in good health when the majority of its citizens spend a fair part of their lives studiously undermining their own health!

The comparison used by the Green Party in its last election manifesto is not inappropriate, as they likened the NHS to a harrassed and increasingly desperate policeman who spends so much time dragging people out of the canal to rescue them from drowning that he has no time to walk up the bank and arrest the criminals and hooligans who keep chucking the people in.

As this book so appositely reminds us, the majority of people in the UK still receive a very high level of health care from the NHS, and there are many countries which look on with no little envy at a service that our own government seems intent on caricaturing as one more appropriate for the Third World.

For all that, the NHS clearly can't cope with the increased pressures on it at this time and although a higher level of funding *might* allow weary administrators to buy in enough elastoplast to cover up the most visible wounds, it would provide no lasting solution.

It must be said that the whole notion of public health is hardly one to stir the emotions, let alone to excite a modicum of political controversy. And that, I fear, is precisely its problem, for it attracts few crusaders and ignites no mass movement. Until that spark is lit, and an awareness of the history, the principles and the practical implication of primary health care runs like brush-fire through the elitist technocracy of modern medicine, I can see no durable solution to the National Health Service's dilemma emerging from within the NHS itself.

The contours of such a solution are sketched out with admirable clarity by Peter Draper and his colleagues in this book. What they have to say is not just clear and informative – it is positively inspirational. As someone who has spent a large part of his life trying to work out the connections between things, and then to explain to bemused, bored and busy people why these connections matter as much if not more than the things themselves, I found myself positively revelling in the web of connections that the many different authors progressively stitch together as each different, notionally separate area is brought into play.

There may be some who will think they're getting more than they asked for as the argument develops, but there is literally no other way of reinventing public health. That challenge has to be confronted even by those who feel most secure and at ease when working to narrow definitions and within segregated categories. Reinventing public health may well entail reinventing human nature!

Though I hesitate to use the word these days, given the confusion it seems to cause, *Health Through Public Policy* would seem to me to be a genuinely 'holistic' book. By emphasising the crucial linkages between health care and economics, trade, politics, international relations, agriculture, transport, energy, planning and freedom of information, it makes whole that which is all too often torn apart.

And in the process, perhaps unwittingly, it provides a framework within which the torn apart shreds of our own bodies, minds and souls could be made whole again. And thereby healed.

Jonathon Porritt

Preface

Health, as we all know, is a possession beyond price. But what is it, where does it come from, how best to guard it? These are the underlying questions addressed in this book. However we personally feel about it, health is more than a biological and psychological state: it is partly a reflection of the wider human condition in all its social, economic and cultural aspects.

The human environment can be more or less favourable; it can enhance well-being or diminish it. When our health is damaged, or we fear it may be, we tend to seek help from the GP, the chemist or the hospital – the 'health' services, which actually cater mainly for the lack of health.

Much less of a misnomer is *public* health. To most health 'consumers' the professions involved in this field normally appear as the dark side of the health moon. While the treatment services are bathed in publicity, glamour and some notoriety, the people responsible for sanitation, food hygiene and catering, safety at work, pollution monitoring, control of epidemics and other preventive measures hit media highspots only over failure in their performance as preventers and watchdogs.

Prevention is better than treatment. It was George Bernard Shaw who said that 'the Medical Officer of Health, unlike practitioners, depends not on the number of people who are ill, but on the number who are well. He is judged as all doctors and treatments should be judged, by the vital statistics of his district' (Preface to *The Doctor's Dilemma*).

But this book takes a wider perspective than the sides of the old arguments between prevention and treatment. Whatever one thinks of the pros and cons of Thatcher rule in the 1980s, few will dispute that the decade has deepened those social and economic inequalities that (equally without effective contradiction) have etched themselves into the statistics not only of employment, nutrition, housing and education, but also those of health. The issue for the next decade is whether struggles to redress society's inbuilt bias which ties the state of people's health to their socio-economic conditions take effect, or whether the rich-poor differential becomes a permanence in the form of a growing underclass of people and families doomed to much worse health than the rest of us.

Peter Draper and his colleagues have cast their net over a broad and diverse field. What has our health got to do with the immoralities of the arms trade to the Third World, with extremist free market ideology recently dominant in Britain, with analysis of different kinds of violence or the threat of mass destruction brought on by nuclear, chemical or other agents of doomsday? Read this book and develop your lateral thinking about health. This need is tragically underscored, as this book goes to press, by the armed conflict in the Gulf, with its immense and escalating violence against people, against the local – and possibly the far wider – environment, and against all hope of enjoying any peace dividend from the ending of the Cold War.

Since classical antiquity people have adopted the personal ideal of *mens sana in corpore sano,* a healthy mind in a healthy body. Today this preoccupation must be extended to the need to secure a healthy body on a healthy planet. The health of individuals is increasingly subject not only to local and regional hazards but also to dangers from other parts of the world, whether from greenhouse contributions or from nuclear accidents that were 'impossible' until they happened. As the 1980s closed, the signs of destruction became clearer, along with the sudden 'Greening' of political parties Left and Right, brought up short after long indifference by incontestable evidence that it is five minutes to midnight on the ecological clock.

The ecological crisis has ushered in a new health challenge, to which the response cannot be individual – whether 'look after yourself' or 'I'm all right'. Neither can ecological health be achieved by East and West on their own, nor by separate continents, neither by the rich of the North nor the poor of the South. Nor can the shift toward destruction be arrested by untrammelled private enterprise organised in groups and blocs. For Brazil's starving landworkers the deforestation which is adulterating the air is their livelihood. Driven by market forces and hunger they are forced to eat their forests. This can be stopped only by international action to provide an alternative livelihood. The politics of conservation and the politics of health protection and promotion are merging into a single set of imperatives.

This is the new emergency and the start of the analysis which for me justifies the scrutiny to which this book exposes the lethal aspects of dominant contemporary thinking about economics and politics. The book's analysis of economic indicators of 'production' and 'growth' underscores the need for an ongoing assessment of the impact of major social and economic activities on people's health and on the environment more generally.

David Player
Director of Public Health
South Birmingham Health Authority

Introduction

Political battles about the National Health Service and glorifications of medical technology focus on treatment rather than prevention. However, as general concern about pollution and other kinds of environmental hazards has grown in Britain and abroad, a complementary approach to traditional public health has emerged. This new public health is Green-sensitive and recognises that the man-made environment in rich and poor countries can adversely affect people's health for socio-economic reasons in addition to the chemical, physical and biological hazards. This book illustrates how today's environment, from agriculture to advertising, from homelessness to energy production, gratuitously damages people's health and it signposts ecological approaches that are in harmony with the World Health Organisation's strategy of promoting healthy public policy as part of its campaign for 'Health For All by the Year 2000'.

The first part of the book (Chapters 1 and 2) surveys this Greening of the new public health and looks at the origins of public health (chiefly in its formative period in Victorian Britain) to evaluate its famous, if flawed and contradictory, legacy and tradition.

Chapters 3, 4 and 5 illustrate how today's environments in very different sectors such as agriculture and food processing, energy, transport and town planning can be health-damaging. These three chapters also consider various enemies of health in the psychic field. These range from the promoters of dangerous and addictive goods like tobacco to the exploitative pushers of armaments and debts onto poor countries. Health-damaging environments are also created by employers providing unsafe and unhealthy conditions of work and by economists and politicians who see unemployment as an economic tool when real levels of wages and public spending are to be cut, ignoring or even denying the health-damaging consequences of involuntary unemployment, as also of bad housing, welfare and nutrition.

The next four chapters (6, 7, 8 and 9) stand back and ask what is happening to the public health watchdogs that are supposed to be protecting us, and they consider underlying political and economic issues affecting public health, including gender politics and the need for new economic concepts and assessments that make sense in ecological terms. In Chapters 10 and 11 suggestions are made about how we might develop a Green-sensitive public health and the last Chapter considers the prospects for a renaissance of public health.

Roughly half the contributors hold different kinds of posts in public health and the other half bring special knowledge and experience of the sectors they write about, from the arms trade to urban and rural planning. Though many of the examples used come from Britain, contributors share a 'one world' perception of the problems which concern North and South in comparable if not identical ways. In other respects, contributors bring different perspectives to bear on the topics they address. Despite the broad canvas, the aim has not been to produce a comprehensive textbook but rather to illustrate how it is useful to look at the health of communities from environmental and policy perspectives. This means that some unarguably important topics for health-promoting policies, like population control, violence, alcohol and illegal drugs, do not get their own sections.

The Green perspective on public health presented in this book was initially developed with Tony Smart and then with colleagues in the Unit for the Study of Health Policy (1975-1984) at Guy's Hospital Medical School, particularly, Gordon Best, Jenny Griffiths, Linda Marks, James Partridge and Jennie Popay. The Trustees of Guy's Hospital gave an invaluable grant to develop the proposals for the Unit and the King's Fund generously gave a five-year founding grant. Also specially supportive in different ways were Jock Anderson, Pat Bolton, James Cornford, John Davoll, John Dennis, Oriole Goldsmith, Gary Grenholm, Miles Hardie, Drummond Hunter, Robert Lindon, Alistair Mackie, Norma McRoy, Teresa Paterson, Hilary Rose and several senior staff of WHO, particularly Halfdan Mahler and Leo Kaprio.

It is a pleasure to acknowledge the help given toward the production of this book and associated broadcasting by a grant from the Health Education Council, organised by its then director general, Dr David Player. Rene Tye, Nina Patel and Debbie Mew provided excellent secretarial support and the librarians of the BMA, the King's Fund Centre and the London Borough of Barnet assisted on many occasions. Many people kindly commented on earlier drafts but special thanks go to Jerry Morris, Alex Scott-Samuel, Ged Moran and Rosemary Hunt. Stanley Harrison generously gave invaluable editorial help and was a source of great encouragement, as were David Player, Christopher Robbins and Marcia Saunders, who was also an outstandingly constructive critic and supporter throughout.

We are grateful to the following for permission to quote: to Professor Colin Spedding for the table on pesticide use and to Greenpeace for the table on North Sea pollution.

Peter Draper

CHAPTER I

A public health approach

Peter Draper

This book is about a new approach to public health, one that is environmental and often Green. This new public health takes a comprehensive view of health hazards in the human environment, from the physical, chemical and biological to the socio-economic. In trying to give effect to new public health the World Health Organisation and countries such as Canada, Australia, Sweden and Norway direct attention to healthy public policy, that is, to ensuring that governmental and non-governmental policies in different sectors such as agriculture, transport and energy are health-promoting or neutral rather than health-damaging. Contributing to the development and implementation of healthy public policies is intrinsically political activity in the general sense but it may or may not harmonise (or clash) with the policies of particular political parties. It is a more fundamental philosophy.

Rediscovering the environment

The core of public health action is avoiding or countering hazards in the environment. This environmental core, the focus of this survey, is concerned with external influences – physical, social and economic – on human well-being. It stands in stark contrast to treatment without regard to prevention and to those kinds of health education (in practice, mainly exhortation and blaming) that are quixotically aimed at changing individual behaviour rather than health-damaging circumstances.

In the past, an environmental approach to health has been strikingly successful. The classic example from the last century is the separation of sewage from drinking water and in this century successes would include the massive reductions in respiratory disease through cleaner air. Yet until recently in Britain and many other countries such an environmental or ecological approach has fallen into neglect, despite a growing understanding – particularly among younger generations – of ecology, that is, of the delicate and complex relationships between living things and their surroundings.

In many countries it took the widespread and lasting radiation effects of the nuclear power plant disaster at Chernobyl to awaken significant anxieties about the environment. Some years before this, however, many people in Nordic and other European countries had become concerned that many of their trees and lakes were either dying or showing signs of damage by acid rain. Indeed, to adapt Ibsen's Dr Stockmann in *An Enemy of the People*, the charge might have been 'the rainwater is poisoned'. In Britain, it took an outspoken health minister (Mrs Edwina Currie) to put public health on the front pages in 1989 by a provocative comment about the scale of salmonella infection in poultry.

Closely linked to environmental concerns in relation to human health, Green politics has emerged in many countries as a minority but influential activity; but with the public's concern about the future of the human environment has reached majority status, particularly since organisations like NASA (the US National Aeronautics and Space Administration) began to comment publicly on the reality of phenomena such as the destruction of the ozone layer and the greenhouse effect. The many connections between general environmental damage and hazards to human health have understandably fostered links between people in and around the new public health and people with Green sensitivities.

What is meant by public health?

To begin this study of new public health we should consider what is meant by the much bigger subject of public health. The often ill-defined term public health normally covers a wide range of activities. A concise and authoritative definition (provided it is understood to include accidents) was recently provided by the first official inquiry into public health in Britain since the 1871 *Report of the Royal Sanitary Commission*:

> the science and art of preventing disease, prolonging life and promoting health through organised efforts of society. (Acheson Report)

A former Scottish chief medical officer's definition (John Brotherston's) has a utilitarian basis and is also succinct: 'The organised application of resources to achieve the greatest health for the greatest number'. An earlier definition by a US authority spelt out the detailed implications of this wider concept as they were seen in WHO circles in 1951:

> Public health is the science and art of
> 1. preventing disease
> 2. prolonging life
> 3. promoting health and efficiency through organised community effort
> 4. a) the sanitation of the environment
>   b) the control of communicable infections
>   c) the education of the individual in personal hygiene
>   d) the organisation of medical and nursing services for the early diagnosis and preventive treatment of disease
>   e) development of the social machinery to ensure everyone a standard of living adequate for the maintenance of health
>
> So organising these benefits so as to enable every citizen to realise his (sic) birthright of health and longevity. (Winslow, 1923 and 1951)

A current and equally authoritative US definition has been provided by a committee of the prestigious Institute of Medicine in its report, *The Future of Public Health*:

> Public health is what we, as a society, do to assure the conditions for people to be healthy. This requires that continuing and emerging threats to the health of the public be successfully countered. These threats include immediate crises, such as the AIDS epidemic; enduring problems, such as the aging of our population and the toxic by-products of a modern economy, transmitted through air, water, soil, or food. (Committee for the Study of the Future of Public Health, p. 19).

Interestingly, this US report goes on to suggest one way in which the word *public* is commonly used in this context by saying 'These and many other problems raise in common the need to protect the nation's health through effective, organized, and sustained efforts *led by the public sector*' (p. 19, my italics). However, elsewhere the report clarifies where it stands when it says the

> mission of public health is addressed by private organizations and individuals as well as by public agencies. But the governmental public

health agency has a unique function: to see to it that vital elements are in place and that the mission is adequately addressed. (p. 7)

In this book 'public health' is used to mean 'concerned with the health of the people' rather than being restricted to the narrower meaning of 'state or local authority health services'. However, in each of the foregoing definitions, through words such as organise, there is a clear expression of political will.

New public health

The sense in which 'new public health' is used in this book is accurately conveyed in the 'Health Promotion Glossary' commissioned by WHO Europe:

> Professional and public concern with the effect of the *total environment* in health.
> *Note* The term builds on the old (especially 19th century) public health which struggled to tackle health hazards in the physical environment (for example, by building sewers). It now includes the socio-economic environment (for example, high unemployment). 'Public health' has sometimes been used to include publicly provided personal health services such as maternal and child care. The term new public health *tends to be restricted to environmental concerns* and to *exclude personal health services, even preventive ones such as immunisation or birth control.* (Nutbeam; my italics)

Immunisation and birth control are of course still essential, but the point is that 'new public health' is not used to mean contemporary, comprehensive public health but rather currently evolving environmental approaches to public health. What then become important are the ways in which the current and future environments are seen and the evolution and implementation of healthy public policies. These topics are now addressed though it should be noted in passing that some authors share these concerns but use 'new public health' in a broader way than the WHO definition quoted (Ashton and Seymour).

In addition it should be noted that there is a sharply contrasted approach to public health, known as *healthism*, that should not be confused with new public health. Healthism sees the achievement of health as the prime object of living. Focused on individuals and on their lifestyles it 'obscures and diminishes the relationships between social and environmental conditions and health' (Nutbeam, p. 119).

Today's and tomorrow's hostile environments

The core of new public health is not only environmental, in recognising new hazards such as damage to the ozone layer (MacKie), it sees these hazards in terms of wider ecological issues. For instance, Halfdan Mahler, the former director-general of WHO, said:

> It has become clear . . . that health is not a private good but a societal, social and individual resource. We are now learning the same about the environment. At the end of the '60s we were actually able to see our planet earth from space for the first time – and for the first time to grasp it as a vulnerable system, whose ecology is something we are responsible for. (Mahler, p. 138)

Making the same point, a recent North American textbook is entitled *Public Health and Human Ecology* (Last).

In some respects, today's environment is of a new kind compared to any previously experienced. It is new because the influences are so much more numerous, more interactive and often more subtle and urgent in the challenges they present. No one who has studied, for instance, the Brundtland Report (World Commission on Environment and Development), or any of the sober and well-documented *State of the World* reports from the Washington-based Worldwatch Institute (Brown), would continue to treat ecological issues in the way in which so many governments and business organisations still do. When Britain's agricultural and industrial revolutions began two centuries ago and greatly increased the output of food and goods, they barely scratched the surface of the ecosystem compared with today's devastation of fields and forests, rivers and oceans, vegetation and fauna, the atmosphere and the soil, and the myopic consumption of finite resources, by governments, banks, agribusiness and industry.

While some ecological problems are now widely recognised, for example, the thinning of the ozone layer, the greenhouse effect, the destruction of tropical rain forests and the indiscriminate use of pesticides, many of the older but no less important problems have yet even to be publicly acknowledged. For instance, and of direct relevance to human nutrition, the massive destruction of fertile soil, which is most dramatic in Africa, cradle of humankind and now a front-line victim of a man-made destruction of the habitat. Two thousand years ago the north of Africa served as the bread-basket of the Roman Empire. Now most of its hundreds of thousands of once cultivated hectares are barren wastes (United Nations Environment Programme, 1987, p.1). An earlier report (1986) from the United Nations Environment Programme recorded that in 1984-6 a 150 kilometre wide belt of the Sahara zone had deteriorated into non-productive desert; in

1976-86, 25 per cent of the 710 million hectares of African pasturelands were lost. The report warned:

> The clock is ticking, an environmental time-bomb. It is now 4.40pm. At the rate of 27 million hectares a year lost to the desert or to zero economic productivity, in a little less than 200 years, at the current rate of desertification, there will not be a single fully productive hectare of land on earth. It will be the earth's midnight . . . We can also be sure that a major socio-economic catastrophe of cataclysmic proportions would engulf the earth long before the last hectare succumbed. We are already feeling the first tremors . . . (p. 92)

There is a substantial overlap between the hostile environment as seen from the perspective of *human* ecology and the kinds of hazards that would be identified on *general* ecological grounds, for instance, in relation to chlorofluorocarbons and the ozone layer. Kickbusch, in an editorial in the WHO-supported quarterly *Health Promotion* (now *Health Promotion International*) summarises some key issues: 'Public health is ecological in perspective, multisectoral in scope and collaborative in strategy', and she offers a new working definition of (new) public health:

> Public health is the science and art of promoting health. It does so based on the understanding that health is a process engaging social, mental, spiritual and physical well-being. It bases its actions on the knowledge that health is a fundamental resource to the individual, the community and to society as a whole and must be supported through sound investments into conditions of living that create, maintain and protect health.

Hostile socio-economic environments

An ecological perspective on human health might also remind us that the environment has micro as well as the more familiar macro characteristics. For instance, we have all been forced to accept that the family can be so hostile to some children that it is lethal. Some of the severest pressures on the micro climate of the family are discussed in Chapter 3.

The new public health also recognises that adverse economic conditions are a highly relevant part of the human environment. In offering an apology for its neglect of this territory, the Acheson Report on public health in England and Wales nonetheless commented:

Nor were we asked to explore the complex social factors underlying health – eg housing, employment, poverty – important though we recognise these to be.

A little earlier the Church of England's inquiry into urban priority areas, *Faith in the City*, went further:

> But if progress is to be made in the larger work of promoting healthy living in urban areas much more attention will have to be paid to the underlying social, economic, housing, environmental and emotional factors which contribute to ill-health. (Canterbury)

The harm that can be done by the economic environment was pinpointed in evidence published in the still impressive report of the 1979 Royal Commission on the National Health Service. The evidence from the William Temple Foundation said:

> It would appear unhelpful to encourage people as individuals to stop smoking, over-indulging in the 'wrong' foods, and leading stressful sedentary lives, when there are evidently so many strong influences encouraging, or even ensuring, that people continue to do these harmful things. (Royal Commission)

The report drew attention to 'a responsibility for preventing illness among its members' that was laid on society. 'Society' has shown a remarkable capacity to digest such rebukes and ignore them. However, people's health needs to be lifted above the scrambles of market forces and declared an area of priority and protection such as defence has long occupied. A coherent and prudent policy for health in agriculture, industry and commerce is essential. Indeed, the Royal Commission also commented:

> To put in perspective what may be accomplished by the NHS, it must be understood that many of the main improvements in the health of the nation have come not from advance in medical treatment but from public health measures, better nutrition and improvements in the economic, social and natural environments.

Because of their importance, socio-economic hazards to health are discussed in Chapters 3, 5, 6 and 9 in relation, for instance, to poverty and parenting, unemployment and stress. Indeed, it would be difficult to overestimate their importance in tackling health inequalities, the generally much worse disease, accident and death rates of the socio-economically disadvantaged. The WHO continues to encourage member countries to address health inequalities, particularly through its 'Health For All by the Year 2000' and 'Healthy Cities' campaigns.

Taking socio-economic factors seriously starts with measuring and monitoring relevant factors when we collect information about people's health. If, for example, we know and record nothing about a family's poverty and their damp and cold housing, however fancy the names we give to the various respiratory diseases that occur, the underlying problems are likely to be overlooked by hospital-based doctors and researchers. The name *social epidemiology* is given to this key and neglected aspect of medical statistics (Scott-Samuel). It is discussed further in Chapter 6.

Access to health-promoting resources, whether food, shelter and clothing, or education, culture, information, or protection by law is strikingly unequal in countries like Britain. Any health 'education' that devolves all the primary responsibility onto the individual fails to identify underlying problems and cannot tackle them competently (Public Health Alliance).

The politics of public health in Britain now particularly arise from the larger governmental strategy of reversing post-war trends in the distribution of general resources, pursued by three Conservative administrations since 1979 and cheered on by so many newspaper word processors. The politics are not simply party-political. The question of redistribution of resources is a controversial one among and within all the major parties. An expanding cross-sectional, cross-class, cross-party range of persons, ages and interests is involved.

We need to reverse our perspectives. The aim should be to integrate the private sector, the market, into the health, safety and welfare sectors. For example, health and safety must – by strict enforcement – come first, as they did not on oil rigs like Piper Alpha in the North Sea, on ferries like the Herald of Free Enterprise at Zeebrugge or in the King's Cross London Underground catastrophe – all in 1987-88. At present the status of health, safety and welfare is that of an adjunct of the business sector – a neglected inspection and repair shop that is under-resourced and often not used or used too late.

The psycho-social environment

The environment has direct influences on people's health and indirect ones that are often less open to analysis. Direct influences include the old scourges of poverty, hunger, infections, inadequate shelter and injuries. Indirect influences are things like the state of local amenities (from shops and sports facilities to public transport), the cash-enforced loneliness of millions of old and not so old people and in particular the effects of fear:

from fear of war to fear of being mugged, of bad neighbours or of returning daily to destructively stressful working conditions, or to the possibilities of the sack.

In the field of mental health many of the practical initiatives to prevent disorder are based on the assumption that socio-economic factors have a major causal or exacerbating influence. A book on prevention in this field reviews rigorously the neglected but extensive and complex literature on environmental factors. It concludes that a reasonable case has already been made for the causal significance of such factors both in first and in recurrent episodes of mental illness. It also examines the harder question of how far preventive methods have succeeded in modifying key social factors. Jennifer Newton's *Preventing Mental Illness* also looks at the way social structures (like parenting and work roles) influence individuals' susceptibility to disorder and recommends that preventive action, to be effective, needs to be aimed at the people most vulnerable to disorders, with voluntary community resources having an essential contribution to make.

Newton quotes Marie Jahoda's distillation of a lifetime's study of unemployment to five main reasons why employment is important: it imposes a time structure on daily activities; it implies regularly shared experiences and contacts with people outside the family; it links an individual to external goals and purposes; it defines aspects of status and identity; and it enforces activity. Newton notes that the definition

> . . . might equally have applied to any of our primary roles. People need a sense of identity and status within a subgroup or culture from a role which requires their active involvement, provides structure to the waking day, provides goals which transcend their own and provides the opportunity for social contact. The extent to which people can obtain these requirements from their primary role, be it worker, parent, student, homemaker or keen amateur darts player, will be related to the presence of depressive symptomatology and recovery from serious psychiatric disorder. (p. 183)

The military environment

If the physical environment is being relentlessly plundered, this organically destructive process is matched by attacks on the human psyche. The problems of the military and civil uses of nuclear energy cast a cloud of literally cosmic insecurity. And if many young people take a dim, fatalistic view of their future, many studies have shown the prevalence of anxieties about a nuclear holocaust (see for instance Solantaus).

WHO has stated that peace, which is more than the absence of war, is a prerequisite for health. For instance, Section X of the famous declaration of Alma-Ata states:

An acceptable level of health for all the people of the world by the year 2000 can be attained through a fuller and better use of the world's resources, a considerable part of which is now spent on armaments and military conflicts. A genuine policy of independence, peace, detente and disarmament could and should release additional resources that could well be devoted to peaceful aims and in particular to the acceleration of social and economic development of which primary health care, as an essential part, should be alloted its proper share. (WHO)

The role of the nuclear arms race in stimulating and distorting powerful market forces is worthy of more study by peace researchers and others. Meanwhile, J. K. Galbraith's chapter 'Economics of the arms race – and after' is a good start. Happily, many medical organisations in a number of countries, like the 'Medical Campaign against Nuclear Weapons' and 'International Physicians for the Prevention of Nuclear War' do a great deal to inform, as does, for instance, the BMA's paperback *The Medical Effects of Nuclear War*. The ugly trade in conventional arms, highly relevant to the 1991 Gulf war and which (in a good year for publicity) might get a TV current affairs programme and a couple of newspaper articles, gets less attention than it deserves: it is discussed in Chapter 5.

Healthier public policies

Acceptance of the fact that people's health is seriously damaged even in industrialised countries by poverty, homelessness and other adverse socio-economic conditions as well as by chemical, biological and physical factors has led WHO, Canada, the Nordic states and other pioneering countries to try to pursue healthy public policies. The Unit for the Study of Health Policy showed how current policies in different fields like transport, agriculture and energy were damaging people's health and how policies outside health services needed to be developed to be health-promoting rather than health-damaging (see for example Draper, Best and Dennis). In an imaginative and amusing paper ostensibly published in AD 2001, Lipton discusses how Britain learned about health-promoting economic development from the Third World and he describes the pursuit of healthy public policy through the creation of a special Cabinet Committee that represented all the sectors, such as agriculture, that shape our environment.

A major landmark in the development of healthy public policy was the publication in 1981 of a book written by an American professor of nursing and public health, Nancy Milio, entitled *Promoting Health Through Public Policy*. The pioneering example that Milio has studied of how there can be progress at a national level if there is enough commitment in the relevant sectors is the slow change over several years to more health-promoting food, farming and fishing policies in Norway (Ziglio). The Norwegian parliament passed a singularly far-sighted Act in 1976 inspired by the twin goals of improving the national diet and trading responsibly with the Third World. For example, basic ideas included reducing the saturated or animal fat content of the Norwegian diet by a number of methods such as replacing some meat by fish and producing leaner meat.

Sweden is a good example of a country that is grappling with healthy public policy in a comprehensive way, including traffic, energy and occupational conditions as well as food (Eklundh and Pettersson). Healthy public policy is not, however, a preserve of rich, egalitarian and healthy Nordic countries. In *Practising Health for All* (Morley et al), some powerful examples are described of outstanding successes of healthy public policies at work in many of the poor countries of the South, for instance, in the Indian State of Kerala, where

despite low per capita income, [Kerala] has dramatically reduced mortality and fertility through emphasising equitable socio-economic and political development.

Six features of healthy public policy

Although healthy public policy is discussed throughout this book because it is the key part of the new public health, six general characteristics should be noted here. First, several sectors are often involved in a given health area. The alcohol industry, for instance, involves catering, employment and transport as well as agriculture and taxation. An Australian health minister commented, 'Health can no longer be pigeon-holed neatly within one government portfolio' (Blewett). This is sometimes described as the need for policy to be 'multisectoral'. The Acheson Report commented on the need for different sectors to co-operate 'to encourage policies which promote and maintain health' (p. 63) and though the committee was hampered by the Prime Minister's decision not to have a Royal Commission or similarly broad-based review it did say

the policies of almost every Government Department can have

implications for health . . . consequently there is a need for effective co-ordination of such policies if health is to be improved. (p. 2)

Second, healthy public policy needs to involve commerce and industry, voluntary organisations and the general public as well as central and local government. Third, health hazards are not confined within national or regional boundaries. As the former director-general of WHO put it:

> National boundaries are a geopolitical fact. But just as health is created largely outside the health sector, so it is created largely across these national boundaries. The winds and viruses will not respect them. The international markets have long transcended them. In health and medicine it is not only the knowledge and the technology that are exported from the industrialised to the developing countries; tobacco, alcohol, pharmaceuticals and consumer goods are also exported. I would add the export of images, ideas about the world and lifestyles – all of which [are] potentially hazardous. (Mahler, p. 133)

Pollution of air and drinking water, seas and forests, respects no political sanctuaries. Chapters 3 and 4 illustrate current hazards in people's environments in industrialised countries with examples which include agriculture and food, energy and transport. The Third World poverty that stems from ill-advised loans and raised interest rates slaughters hundreds of thousands of children and adults each year in different countries, as discussed in Chapter 5.

The fourth feature of healthy public policy to consider here is that the aim is to be educational and persuasive rather than dictatorial or puritanical. It is easy to misrepresent new public health as some kind of medical megalomania with the health sector apparently trying to run the world! Rather, the aim is to get the substantial health impacts of different sectors such as agriculture or transport taken seriously so that, for example, the health sector is not urging people to consume less animal fat while the agricultural sector is bribing farmers to produce fatter cattle and creamier milk. Where enemies of public health (such as tobacco, alcohol and other drug pushers) refuse to act in the public interest, legal or financial pressures are necessary, but this fourth feature has been aptly summarised in the phrase 'Make the healthy choices the easier choices'.

The fifth feature is that effective work for healthy public policy does not need to be formal in the sense of holding formal meetings or involving other organisations, whether official, voluntary or industrial-commercial. Indeed, quite as important as the local, regional, national and international levels that we have been considering are initiatives that occur in small communities, for instance, in a block of flats or among parents from a local school to tackle problems in their micro-environments such as unsafe play areas or racist attacks. These are often called 'community health initiatives' and in Britain there is an organisation to help them to exchange ideas and information and sometimes to help them get financial and other material help – National Community Health Resource.

The sixth and last feature is that healthy public policy is intrinsically political but not party-political. Public health – the health of the people – is inextricably political, whether a country has a formal and explicit policy for public health or not. However, supporters and opponents of public health can be found in each and every party – though anyone who was so conservative as to be totally opposed to all change or so anarchist or market-worshipping as to oppose all regulations would find it exceedingly difficult to accept public health strategies and support efforts to reduce the avoidable health hazards in the environment.

Furthermore, while supporters and opponents of public health are found across the party spectrum, it would be misleading not to point out that many supporters cluster in its Green, Orange, Red and Red-Green bands. For instance, the Liberal Party published a far-sighted report about healthy public policy which had the neat title *Health is Everything*. Although public health requires changes in legislation and a budget (the route to which normally lies through elections and party strife), health is a wider concern than parties – based on conflicting interest groups and ideologies – can represent or encompass. We are talking about health for all and all for health. This is politics with a difference, transcending party lines.

The politics of public health

So how should the non-party politics of this environmental and policy part of public health be defined? Most broadly, perhaps, as a fundamental philosophy and collaboration to maximise the influences operating to promote health and minimise those tending to damage it. If models are needed, analogous cross-party and cross-class movements exist, such as the women's movement, Friends of the Earth, the anti-apartheid organisations and those for nuclear disarmament. These all promote causes that are intensely political but they avoid ties to particular parties.

Public health, like the NHS, has often been kicked between Left and Right goalposts. In Left thinking, however, there are signs that warfare on sectarian, party lines about ecological and public health issues is beginning to be seen as counter-productive. Steve Watkins, a contributor to this volume, notes that it is no longer in the interests of the Left to try to disturb the 'non-political' standing of the medical profession. However, before we become complacent we should remember the many successes of Mrs Thatcher's and President Reagan's administrations in moving the goal posts to the Right and so putting many public services into controversial territory if not abolishing them.

The word 'political' in current British usage is not only assumed to imply 'party', it is loaded with other negative connotations. Used in discussions of health policy, 'political' often connotes sordid vested interest, bias or manipulation. Leaving aside the anomaly of such views co-existing with feelings of pride in democracy, the plain fact is that politics is, has been and will be, dirty and clean, principled and unprincipled. Overt political involvement in contemporary Britain, irrespective of party (except perhaps the Green Party), is commonly regarded as some kind of disreputable deviance. Such nastiness as there clearly is will not be confronted if citizens decide to boycott public business. How different were the politics of the privileged Athenians of Periclean times, for whom an intelligent interest in their *polis* was a duty as well as a right.

Other political aspects of public health and the economic factors that often cause them to emerge are discussed in Chapters 7 and 8 respectively.

The NHS and public health

Not since the inception of the NHS over forty years ago has the relationship with public health ever been more than a peripheral one, whatever the rhetoric. Indeed, it has become a common jibe that the NHS is really the National Sickness Service. We argue for recognition of the *complementarity* of public health and treatment services as a sounder basis for tackling the teeming problems of the illness service. The failure to comprehend this complementarity is starkly demonstrated each time a minister ignores greatly increased poverty, involuntary unemployment, homelessness and other health hazards over the last decade and brags that the NHS is 'treating more patients than ever', clearly believing that this is some kind of *health* achievement!

The greater role for public health that is needed should not come at the expense of the sickness service. Common sense rightly sees good treatment and care services as an essential part of a civilised society and modern scientific medicine has more to offer people than it currently does in Britain. Spending on health care in most other industrialised countries is significantly higher. Sweden and the US, for example, have for years allocated a slice of the national cake (GNP or GDP) *half as big again* as the British 6 per cent or so. Contrary to the long running disinformation campaigns of governments and most of the tabloids, the NHS has suffered not only low, but unpredictable funding. That underfunding led to the staff shortages and ward closures in 1988/91, for example. Instead of getting a little more of our taxes, the NHS got a glossy government White Paper and a propaganda bombardment about yet another Conservative management reorganisation – their fourth. The line was that NHS (i.e. public) health care was seriously flawed despite informed opinion internationally. Also, by ignoring the experience of staff, the government rendered the management experience of thousands of doctors, nurses and other staff worthless, indeed, something to be steamrollered in the way management treats industrial workers when it is going to impose contentious changes.

The NHS not only delivers a staggering volume of treatment, care and some preventive services to nearly everyone, it is an outstandingly cost-effective example of such a system. Mainly because it does not have to pay expensive insurance bureaucracies, its administrative overheads have been remarkably low (about 5-6 per cent) compared with those of insurance-based health care, for instance in the US (which groan away at well over 20 per cent). The fact that such achievements are not widely known says much about our national press and government propaganda.

Anyone who doubts the value of the NHS should visit the US and see hospital emergency rooms, follow a few ambulances or stay in a community that announces as you enter, 'This town needs a doctor'. That is not to suggest there are no problems in the NHS, but rather that the basic principles and structure were sound. Real progress should have come from building on the solid foundations and part of that development should have been public health. The government's insistence on developing an 'internal market' within the NHS from 1991 is not only preparing the ground for extensive privatisation, it is also a recipe for soaring accountancy and other bureaucratic overheads not contributing to clinical care.

Some NHS staff carry out valuable tasks which are usually seen as public health activities. These tend to be tasks of surveillance (such as checking children's development), advice on birth control and other important preventive interventions such as immunisation. They usually take place in health clinics, centres and GPs' surgeries rather than in hospitals. These services prevent or greatly reduce much human misery which would otherwise occur through infections, unwanted pregnancies or correctable development problems.

Accidents and illnesses are also prevented by a 'greater public health team' outside the NHS, consisting most obviously of environmental health officers, but also of many other kinds of workers from those who maintain sewers to those concerned with health and safety at workplaces of all kinds. Less obviously, many other people contribute, for instance, all those who work for road safety, like teachers, health educators or good publicans who try to keep driving and alcohol separate, and people who provide good rail and bus services which reduce the volume of road traffic.

Why should it be wise to try to reclaim or reinvent public health in Britain or elsewhere if there are already so many people doing useful work? The answer we see is that despite all this effort, there are many activities in agriculture and food processing, in industrial and commercial organisations like tobacco firms, breweries and advertising agencies that too often still seriously threaten many people's health and frequently children's in particular. Furthermore, as we shall see in Chapters 6 and 7, the watchdogs of public health and safety can be starved, can lose their teeth or be muzzled.

Conclusion

Competitive games between preventers and treaters, between environmentalists and practitioners of modern or western scientific medicine, are inherently futile. Health, like society more generally, needs to develop more co-operative patterns. Much more could be done in most countries to develop public health and prevent avoidable suffering. There is no room, though, for vague fantasies about abolishing the need for treatment services through some kind of perfection of public health, however effective and efficient prevention becomes.

Human health is not to be perfected. A well-known WHO definition of health is 'a state of complete physical, mental and social well-being, and not merely the absence of disease or infirmity'. Nobody enjoys such complete well-being and the definition has often been criticised for being utopian – and impossible to use as a basis for measurement. Nevertheless, a Swedish study finds that the definition is 'a very valuable signpost indicating the direction of the health objective . . . it expresses a value, namely the *experience* of health as the main consideration rather than the objectively measurable state' (Lagergren et al, p. 25). The point is that health is about mental or spiritual well-being as well as acceptable biochemical and other tests.

If complete well-being is utopian, the broader concept of wholeness in people is not and its ingredients are increasingly seen to range from the largest – like the outlook for world peace – to the smallest, like a good night's sleep. *Faith in the City* added the support of the Anglican church:

The church needs to promote a broader understanding of the meaning of health. This must be concerned with more than the absence of disease. It must concern the Biblical concept of Shalom and wholeness: for the care we take of the quality as well as the length of people's lives. (Canterbury)

Traditional approaches to health care, based on self-care by the individual and professional treatment of serious illness, require redefinition. On the one hand, good clinical treatment and care must remain a right in any civilised society. On the other hand, a development of prevention and health promotion through ecological approaches is urgent.

REFERENCES

Acheson Report, *Public Health in England: The Report of the Committee of Inquiry into the Future Development of the Public Health Function* (London, 1988).

J. Ashton and H. Seymour (eds.), *The New Public Health: The Liverpool Experience* (Milton Keynes, 1988).

N. Blewett, 'Health for all Australians', *Positive Health*, 7 (1988).

BMA, *The Medical Effects of Nuclear War: The Report of the British Medical Association's Board of Education and Science* (Chichester, 1983).

L.R. Brown, *State of the World: A Worldwatch Institute Report on Progress Toward a Sustainable Society* (London, 1988).

Canterbury, *Faith in the City: The Report of the Archbishop of Canterbury's Commission on Urban Priority Areas* (London, 1985).

Committee for the Study of the Future of Public Health, *The Future of Public Health* (Washington, 1988).

H. Crawley, 'Promoting Health Through Public Policy', *Health Promotion*, 2, 2 (1987).

P. Draper, G. Best and J. Dennis, 'Health and Wealth', *Royal Society of Health Journal*, 97 (1977).

B. Eklundh and B. Pettersson, 'Health Promotion Policy in Sweden: Means and Methods in Intersectoral Action', *Health Promotion*, 2, 2 (1987).

J.K. Galbraith, 'Economics of the Arms Race – and After', in R. Adams and S. Cullen (eds.), *The Final Epidemic: Physicians and Scientists on Nuclear War* (Chicago, Educational Foundation for Nuclear Science, 1981).

I. Kickbusch, 'Approaches to an Ecological Base for Public Health', *Health Promotion*, 4, 4 (1989).

M. Lagergren, L. Lundh, M. Orkan and C. Sanne, *Time to Care: A Report Prepared for the Swedish Secretariat for Future Studies* (Oxford, 1984).

J. Last, *Public Health and Human Ecology* (East Norwalk, Connecticut, 1987).

Liberal Party, *Health is Everything* (Hebden Bridge, 1985).

M. Lipton, 'From Protective Health to National Recovery?', *Institute of Development Studies Bulletin*, 9, 2 (1977).

R.M. MacKie and M.J. Rycroft, 'Health and the Ozone Layer: Skin Cancers May Increase Dramatically', *British Medical Journal*, 297 (1988).

H. Mahler, 'Keynote Address, Second International Conference on Health Promotion', *Health Promotion*, 3, 2 (1988).

N. Milio, *Promoting Health Through Public Policy* (Philadelphia, 1981).

D. Morley, J. Rohde and G. Williams (eds.), *Practising Health for All* (Oxford, 1983), p. 64.

National Community Health Resource, *A New Voice for Health* (London, NCHR, 1988).

J. Newton, *Preventing Mental Illness* (London, 1988).

D. Nutbeam, 'Health Promotion Glossary', *Health Promotion*, 1, 1 (1986).

Public Health Alliance, *A Charter for Public Health* (PHA, Room 204, Snow Hill House, 10-15 Livery Street, Birmingham B3 2PE, 1987).

Royal Commission on the National Health Service, *Report* (London, 1979).

A. Scott-Samuel, 'Building the New Public Health: A Public Health Alliance and a New Social Epidemiology', in C.J. Martin and D.V. McQueen (eds.), *Readings for a New Public Health* (Edinburgh, 1989).

T. Solantaus, 'Hopes and Worries of Young People in Three European Countries', *Health Promotion*, 2, 1 (1987).

United Nations Environment Programme, *Annual Report* (Nairobi, UNEP, 1986).

United Nations Environment Programme, *The State of the World Environment* (Nairobi, UNEP, 1987).

S. Watkins, *Medicine and Labour: The Politics of a Profession* (London, 1987).

C.E.A. Winslow, *The Cost of Sickness and the Price of Health* (Geneva, WHO, 1951). Based on the author's earlier definition in *The Evolution and Significance of the Modern Public Health Campaign* (New Haven, 1923).

World Commission on Environment and Development, *Our Common Future* (The Brundtland Report) (New York, WCED, 1987).

WHO, *Report of the International Conference on Primary Health Care, Alma-Ata, USSR* (Geneva, WHO, 1978), Health for All series.

E. Ziglio, '"Uncertainty" in Health Promotion: Nutrition Policy in Two Countries', *Health Promotion*, 1, 3 (1986).

FURTHER READING

Nancy Milio, *Promoting Health Through Public Policy*, 2nd ed. (Ottawa, Canadian Public Health Association, 1986). A classic. WHO's European officer for health promotion has gone on record as saying that this rich and pioneering book has 'heavily influenced . . . thinking on health promotion policy' within WHO.

J. Ashton and H. Seymour, *The New Public Health: The Liverpool Experience* (Milton Keynes, 1988). This lively and useful study is rooted in real engagement with an English region and WHO's 'Healthy Cities' project.

Claudia Martin and David McQueen, *Readings for a New Public Health* (Edinburgh, 1989). Another useful collection, including for instance Alex Scott-Samuel's well-documented chapter on building the new public health and developing a new social epidemiology.

Research Unit in Health and Behavioural Change, *Changing the Public Health* (Chichester, 1989). An interdisciplinary group with the social sciences appropriately dominant. Clearly written and stimulating.

Stephen Farrow, *The Public Health Challenges* (London, 1987). In contrast with the previous volume, medical perspectives – apart from Jane Lewis, an important proviso. Published for the Faculty of Community Medicine, now the Faculty of Public Health Medicine.

Lorenz Ng and Devra Davis, *Strategies for Public Health: Promoting Health and Preventing Disease* (New York, 1981). Twenty-six concise chapters from different disciplines on a range of mainly still-relevant topics such as the logistical problems of toxicological tests (Chapter 9). The publisher's blurb arguably claims that the book 'is the first reference of its kind to question the assumption of fixed levels of sickness or pathology . . .'.

John Last, *Public Health and Human Ecology* (East Norwalk, Connecticut, 1987). An enlightened 400-page student textbook from an Australian professor of public health who works in North America.

Godfrey Gunatilleke, *Intersectoral Linkages and Health Development: Case Studies in India (Kerala State), Jamaica, Norway, Sri Lanka and Thailand* (Geneva, WHO,

1984), WHO Offset Publication No 83. The state of some national and international arts at the beginning of the 1980s.

Special aspects

Alwyn Smith and Bobbie Jacobson (eds.), *The Nation's Health: A Strategy for the 1990s* (Oxford, 1988). A heroic review of the possibilities for prevention in Britain as judged from epidemiological data around the mid-1980s. The political aspects were fatal for this 'Independent Multidisciplinary Committee' and the five sponsoring organisations. The report says, apparently without realising (or admitting) how many questions it was begging, that its technocratic approach 'will also enable us to set *realistic targets which are achievable in policy terms*' (p. 237, my italics). Homelessness gets four lines.

Brian Inglis, *The Diseases of Civilisation: An Indictment of Traditional Methods of Medical Treatment and a Plea for a Completely New Approach* (London, 1981). A much better introduction to critiques of modern scientific medicine than Ivan Illich's.

Robert Nisbet, *The Social Philosophers: Community and Conflict in Western Thought* (London, 1974). The 64-page chapter on the evolution and thinking of ecological communities – which ranges from St Francis through Sir Thomas More and his *Utopia* to Proudhon and Kropotkin – has remarkable relevance to the social philosophies for healthy public policies.

Hilary Burrage, 'Epidemiology and Community Health: A Strained Connection?', *Social Science and Medicine,* 25, 8 (1987). A cogent critique of epidemiology from a sociological perspective.

The January 1991 edition of *Public Health* was dedicated to Alwyn Smith to mark his retirement. The papers by Boddy, Jefferys, Jacobson and Eskin particularly give an excellent introduction to the perspective of British epidemiology and public health up to the end of the 1980s.

CHAPTER 2

The origins of public health: concepts and contradictions

Eric Ross

*Societies that we call primitive usually took the social character
of the human condition for granted and understood how
individual health depended on it. In contrast, this chapter
traces the rise of a savagely individualist ethos in the heyday of
capitalist industrialisation that predominantly interpreted high
rates of illness, accidents and death among the poor as signs of
personal inadequacy. This put a stamp of contradiction on
Britain's pioneering public health tradition, whose proponents
in different ways were Jeremy Bentham, Edwin Chadwick and
Herbert Spencer. A persistent dissident challenge, from doctors
like Charles Hall in Britain, Johann Peter Frank and Rudolf
Virchow in Germany, and William Gorgas and Joseph
Goldberger in America, is traced. The chapter calls for this
alternative tradition to be reclaimed, as the basis for a new
model 'political ecology of health'.*

'Public health' emerges

The concept of 'public health' is largely a product of the last century and the
social crisis created by the epidemic diseases that ravaged the human
landscape of urban industrial capitalism. But, because the geography of
infection and death reflected the class character of nineteenth-century
society, it was a concept which reflected not only the impact of epidemic
events, but the contradictions of divergent class interests.

Before pursuing some of the implications of this, it is salutary to suggest
that the very emergence of an idea of public health, still contradictory and
contentious today, belies the normal cultural experience of most preindustrial peoples (and by extension most of human history) who have

generally taken for granted the fundamental tenet of public health practice, that individual and collective health are indivisible.

Anthropologists have long been aware of the fact that in state-less societies it is rare to find a distinctive field of knowledge equivalent to western medicine; questions of disease are commonly inseparable from the condition of society as a whole. As one writer has noted of the Foré people of highland New Guinea, 'Beliefs about the etiology of disease are statements about the nature of existence, explanations of why things happen as they do' (Lindenbaum, p. 56). For the same reason, among the Tapirapé Indians of Eastern Brazil the responsibilities of a shaman were not restricted merely to narrow matters of obvious illness. According to Charles Wagley, 'The Tapirapé depended on their shamans to control the dangerous spirit world, to remove danger from first fruits, to predict the future, to bring spirits of children to their prospective parents, and to cure the ill. In all life situations where chance or the unpredictable figured, the Tapirapé depended markedly upon their shamans' (p. 195).

This absence of a precise, mechanical boundary between the individual and society or between society and nature in the matter of physical or moral well-being, is not entirely alien to western tradition. The ancient Greeks respected the susceptability of the human body to environmental conditions and regarded illness as a disturbance of a natural equilibrium between the individual's external and internal environments. Many of the principles of Greek thinking about health and illness proved resilient and enduring, particularly the notion of bodily humours whose proper balance was essential for individual health. Recast by medieval society, many of these ideas survived in English medical thought into the nineteenth century. But by then they had become a dogma, the limits of which were sorely taxed by the profound social, economic and epidemiological changes then engulfing European society.

As such, they dominated the thinking of major figures in the sanitary reform movement – individuals such as Edwin Chadwick and Florence Nightingale – who regarded disease as the product of foul air and 'miasmas'. Before the contagion model became fully established in the second half of the nineteenth century, this causal framework contained sufficient ambiguity to allow epidemic diseases to be susceptible to some remedy yet able to be regarded as a metaphysical disorder or a moral judgement. Thus, the arrival of cholera in the US in 1832 was widely interpreted 'as an inevitable result of the debilitating physical effect of transgressing [God's] physical and moral laws' (Rosenberg, p. 258). The opportunity to attribute disease to the moral deficiencies of its victims proved far too useful in certain quarters to yield readily to the new insights of epidemiological science, and it gave to much of public health thinking a certain messianic flavour (Wohl, pp. 6-9).

Medicine, which entered the nineteenth century still largely characterised by a medieval pharmacopia, was often little more than a compound of superstition, quackery and wishful thinking (Young). Yet it was being overtaken by events. The swift transformation of villages into factory towns and cities, the crowding of families of workers into dank, airless housing built often on speculation by absentee landlords, the pollution of water by factory effluent and human waste – all these created new environmental hazards to which medical practitioners often seemed incapable of reacting. Some, like the surgeon William Moss of Liverpool, seemed on the one hand prisoners of medieval thinking and, on the other, perhaps a bit too circumspect and politic to exercise their independent critical judgement. In 1784, Moss discussed the problem of the open sewers which traversed one of the poorer districts of the city and noted:

> The common sewer . . . has been generally esteemed an addition to their unhealthfulness. The disagreeable smell, which sometimes issues from it, chiefly creates this alarm; which is more imaginary than real; as the simple decay of any substance, whether animal or vegetable, is not so baneful to the human constitution as is commonly supposed. (p. 43)

But, while Moss was arguing that the 'fixed air' produced by the fermentation of waste was actually a palliative, the well-to-do were obviously unconvinced and preferred to move their residences to more salubrious locations farther out of the city.

Momentous advance – long resisted

This is not to say that there was no movement on the medical front. Perhaps the most momentous was the development of innoculation, as a means of preventing infectious disease. The practice was, in fact, a comparatively old one outside Europe and seems to have been incorporated into the repertoire of European folk-medicine by the early eighteenth century. The disease most frequently associated with innoculation, or variolation as it was also known, was smallpox, one of the most dreaded illnesses and one which inflicted death and disability on a scathing scale. But, until the late 1700s, innoculation was not without dangers, as it depended on transmission of the live smallpox germ itself (Chase, pp. 44-5). It was not until Edward Jenner, a Gloucestershire physician, developed a method of vaccination against smallpox which refined a rural practice of acquiring immunity through infection with the more benign disease of cowpox, that a means of eliminating the scourge of smallpox actually arose. Had the concept of 'public health' been a clear and uncontentious one, Jenner's method of vaccination might have been promptly and widely implemented. But, despite the view taken by many doctors (though not by all) that it was not only safe but effective, the idea of government-sponsored low-cost or free smallpox vaccination made little headway in Britain during the nineteenth century (Chase, pp. 63-4). Here, as well as in other parts of Europe and in the US, there was surprisingly substantial opposition, principally on political and religious grounds, to a public health measure which had been proven to be medically sound.

Resistance to such medical advance came from several directions. England was a class-stratified society, characterised by profound disparities in property ownership and income. In the late eighteenth and early nineteenth centuries, these differences grew as rural enclosures signified the triumph of commercial agriculture and as cottage industries were swept aside by centralised, intensive industrial production. Among the dramatic consequences of these transformations was the rise of dense urban concentrations of working people in overcrowded, unhygienic living conditions which were breeding grounds for virulent infections (Harris and Ross, pp. 113-5). Diseases such as tuberculosis, typhoid and smallpox were not new, but the industrial revolution created environmental conditions in which they could flourish.

It is incontrovertible that the growth of industrial towns induced rising mortality. This mortality was notable in two particular respects. First, it was increasingly concentrated among young children (Harris and Ross, p. 115); and secondly, it disproportionately affected the working class. While industrial life granted the middle class a flourishing lifestyle, marked by improved housing, decent diet and remunerative and unexhausting work, the factory system, with its onerous labour and cycles of employment and redundancy, meant low wages, poor housing, inadequate food – all life-threatening – to the working class. Industrialisation exacerbated all the pre-existent disparities in material well-being, and thereby deepened the class-determined nature of health and survival itself.

There were many who could only regard the growing immiseration of the working class in terms of their personal failings, who could never see in their smoking or drinking a modest refuge from daily struggles but only the symptoms of moral inadequacy. Writing at the end of the eighteenth century, before the full impact of industrialisation had even been felt, Sir Frederick Morton – much like Edwina Currie almost two centuries later – had written: 'There seems to be just reason to conclude that the miseries of the poor arise less from the scantiness of their income . . . than from their own improvidence and unthriftiness'.

But, to others, including some medical practitioners, a more intimate experience suggested that the poverty and ill-health of individuals were essentially social products. One notable example was Charles Hall, a doctor from the west of England, whose book *The Effects of Civilisation on the People in European States*, published in 1805, anticipated a number of important ideas in the work of Marx and Engels. A lifetime of medical work led Hall to conclude that 'the greater mortality among the poor can only be owing to the differences in the manner in which they are supplied with the necessities of life'. Their plight was the result of scarcity and deprivation, not of laziness or divine will, and it therefore required for its amelioration a total alteration of how society was organised, of how goods were produced and wealth apportioned.

The Malthusian philosophy

In an appendix to his book Hall reserved special criticism for the writings of the Reverend Thomas Malthus, whose pamphlet on population (1798) had become a rallying point for opponents of public obligation to the poor. In the Malthusian view, poverty was the natural result of disparities between resources and population. While Malthus recognised that 'in the history of every epidemic it has invariably been observed that the lower classes of people, whose food was insufficient, and who lived crowded together in small and dirty houses, were the principal victims', his appeal to both gentry and industrialist was that he chose to absolve society of either blame or responsibility for such associations and to hold the poor – and especially what he viewed as their propensity for excessive breeding – personally accountable for their situation. He also regarded their death-rate from poverty, malnutrition and disease as the principal means by which their excess numbers – and thus their potential threat to social stability – were reduced. As such, he was particularly opposed to medical innovators such as Jenner, 'those benevolent, but mistaken men, who have thought they were doing a service to mankind' but were only confounding the course of nature (quoted in Chase, p. 56).

The Malthusian philosophy – so antithetical to any concept of 'public health' – was born out of the needs and motives of the English ruling class in the new circumstances of nineteenth-century capitalism. Among these initially was the wish to sweep away what many regarded as the antiquated and costly remnants of an earlier generation's notion of social concern, in particular the Poor Law system derived from Elizabethan legislation. Three years before the publication of Malthus' *Essay*, a meeting of magistrates, clerics and others at Speenhamland in Berkshire gave its name to a widespread effort to modify the old system of parish relief, instituting a new arrangement which ostensibly geared relief to the cost of bread but in fact created 'a universal system of pauperism' (Hammond and Hammond, p. 164; cf. Hobsbawm and Rudé, pp. 47ff). The so-called Speenhamland system neither alleviated the most fundamental structural problems of poverty nor satisfied those who believed, with Malthus, that relief generally was wasteful and counterproductive.

The Elizabethan Poor Law, of course, had never been entirely a charitable measure. Promulgated at a time when land clearances were creating a vagabond army of the unemployed (Morton, pp. 165-8), it was meant chiefly to police the movements of the poor by restricting pubic assistance to their home parishes. Nonetheless, by the early nineteenth century, it had come to represent the idea that the poor had an entitlement to some form of social support (Beer, p. 85). Speenhamland had not done anything to reverse that, nor had it helped – as the capitalist class wished – to increase the mobility of labour (Morton, p. 396). Substantive reform of the system of public assistance remained on the agenda of the ruling class and, with the help of Malthus' writings, was finally achieved in 1834 with new legislation which 'set the seal on unfettered free trade in the labour market' (Dobb, p. 275). Workers could either 'get on their bikes' or face confinement in the Poor House.

Chadwick's sanitary reform

Malthus' ideas were shaped by and in turn influenced other writers and thinkers, including the formidable Jeremy Bentham, the founder of Utilitarianism (Morton and Tate, p. 73). Bentham was a friend of the Reverend Joseph Townsend, whose *Dissertation on the Poor Laws* (1786) was a major source of many of Malthus' own ideas (Langer, pp. 669-70) and whose personal credo was neatly summed up in his observation that 'wretchedness has increased in proportion to the efforts made to relieve it' (quoted in Chase, p. 55). One of Bentham's chief acolytes, a man equally imbued with the Malthusian temper, was the barrister Edwin Chadwick, who is widely credited with being the pillar of the British movement for sanitary reform and a founder of the field of public health.

Chadwick, however, embodied the contradictions which were embraced by the concept of public health in the nineteenth century. As one of the authors of the Poor Law Amendment Act of 1834, he is acknowledged to have played a singular role in translating Malthusian doctrine into practice. By abolishing outdoor relief and making conditions within workhouses so miserable that virtually anyone would despair of the thought of entering one, the new law – a model of Thatcherite legislation – at once reduced public expenditure and guaranteed a reserve of labour intimidated by fear of life in the so-called 'bastilles'.

As Morton has noted,

The administration of the Act was deliberately removed as far as possible from popular control by the appointment of three virtually irresponsible Commissioners, the 'three Kings of Somerset House', who became for a whole decade, together with their Secretary, Edwin Chadwick, the most detested men in England. (p. 397)

This was not entirely unreasonable. Within two years of the passage of the new Poor Law, Chadwick had authored his *Police Report* of 1839 which helped to establish the English constabulary. By his own admission, among the main purposes of the police were to subdue opposition to the operation of the new Poor Law and to protect the interests of industrialists. In both cases, this meant utilising the police to suppress the activities of trade unions and other working class movements such as Chartism (Finer, pp. 178-80).

In Chadwick's view – and he was scarcely alone in this – the defense of civil order clearly took precedence over matters of health; indeed, his interest in health emerged out of his Benthamite preoccupation with social efficiency and stability. It was in the course of their work on the Poor Law Commission, in fact, that Chadwick and his colleagues began to turn their attention to the issue of preventable urban sickness and mortality, for what guided their thinking was less a compassionate idea of health *per se* than the utilitarian view that 'The expenditure necessary to the adoption and maintenance of measures of prevention would ultimately amount to less than the cost of the disease now constantly engendered' (quoted in Frazer, p. 31).

By 1842, Chadwick had authored his famous *Report on an Inquiry into the Sanitary Conditions of the Labouring Population of Great Britain*. Along with his subsequent work as Commissioner of the General Board of Health from 1848 to 1854, it proved of immense significance in helping to fight for improvements in urban environmental health services, including sewage and water supply. But what is strikingly obvious about the 1842 *Report* – though perhaps not surprising in light of Chadwick's political and social views – is that, despite its publication in the name of the Poor Law Commission, it made virtually no reference to unemployment or low wages, no inferences or suggestions about the economic dimension of health. This, however, was not unusual among public health advocates of the day. In 1848 Dr Hector Gavin, lecturer in forensic medicine and public health at Charing Cross Hospital, published a study of conditions in Bethnal Green in London's East End which managed not only to neglect the subject of unemployment, but to dismiss the notion that poor diet might contribute to the area's high mortality.

By mid-century, successive epidemics of cholera and typhoid were features of urban industrial life in Europe and the US, and it was these which stimulated the concern which eventuated in the sanitary reform movement. But it was a concern that contained an ideological bias. After all, tuberculosis was a far greater killer (Tesh, p. 322), but it was a disease which disproportionately affected the poor. In contrast, the water-borne diseases such as typhoid and cholera were much less likely to respect class boundaries and so represented the kind of threat which demanded action at the societal level.

The perspective of the sanitary reformers such as Chadwick and Florence Nightingale (who came to prominence during the Crimean War when more British soldiers died of infection than of bullets) was also dictated, as I have suggested earlier, by their disbelief in the theory of contagion. Neither ever accepted the existence of pathogenic organisms, both instead based their efforts entirely on the view that disease was the product of filth and smells (Chase, pp. 104-7; McKeown, 1979, p. 160), a view which emphasised the problem of water-borne diseases. This was something of an advance on the stance of Dr Moss of Liverpool and, to a large extent, it freed their work of the kind of intellectual complications that might easily have retarded the development of practical public services. As a result, an array of sanitary measures – improved water supplies, better sewage removal, cleaner streets – helped virtually to eliminate diseases such as cholera and typhoid in a comparatively short space of time.

Yet, as W.M. Frazer, medical officer of health in post-war Liverpool, remarked,

> the virtual suppression of epidemics and an appreciable reduction in
> death-rates only went a short way towards the solution of the problem
> of ensuring and maintaining the health of the population. Much still
> remained to be accomplished while the greater part of the working-class
> population was ill-housed, poorly fed and illiterate. (pp. 158-9)

Bentham and Chadwick – conservative forces

But, at a time of conflicting theories of disease causation (Tesh), Chadwick's faith in the disease-causing properties of miasmas had commended itself in part because it had not implied the need for the kind of social or economic change that would have helped to redress such structural problems. His analytical convictions were progressive to the extent that they asserted an environmental component of disease, but they were limited in turn by a view of the environment which was instrumental rather than social. As such the Public Health Act of 1848, in large part a result of Chadwick's efforts, not only effectively enshrined the miasma theory in law – only a year before John Snow set forth his views on the transmission of cholera – but focused attention on a strictly delimited aspect of disease which excluded any overtly political or economic dimension by defining it essentially as a problem of engineering.

As a result, the principal successes in the field of health in the nineteenth century were essentially triumphs not of medical practice or scientific theory (McKeown, 1979, 1983; Rosen), but of efforts to reorganise aspects of the human environment in a largely mechanical sense. In practical terms, this had undeniable and significant effects on health. But preoccupation with sanitary measures barely permitted the elaboration of the concept of public health as a means of addressing or remedying fundamental problems of social justice. One important reason for this, it must be said, was that the utilitarian thinking which inspired reformers such as Chadwick was implicitly conservative. Its concern for the threat that epidemic disease represented to social order and economic productivity (cf. Tesh, p. 339) made it particularly congenial to the interests of the middle class, but necessarily restricted its perspective on society as a whole.

It had an additional appeal to a middle class constituency, and that was its moral view of the poor and the causes of social disorder. While Chadwick's assumption that disease was an effect of 'atmospheric impurity' effectively dissociated the epidemiological process from the structural determinants of poverty, it possessed the additional merit of sustaining the Victorian idea that the physical conditions in which the poor lived, rather than the political economy which governed their means of employment, were at the root of crime and allied threats to middle class life. As Chadwick himself wrote in 1874,

> how much of rebellion, of moral depravity and of crime has its root in
> physical disorder and depravity . . . The fever nests and seats of
> physical depravity are also the seats of moral depravity, disorder and
> crime with which the police have the most to do.

Thus, Chadwick and his associates regarded their efforts not primarily as a means of improving the health of the poor but rather as a practical means of achieving social stability by implementing the Victorian view that cleanliness would bring the poor closer to godliness. In contrast, a perspective on public health which placed greater emphasis on political and economic reform would have seemed to threaten the very stability to which they aspired. As such, it would have been antithetical to the interests of capital and the demands of middle class morality.

know. Many of the additives permitted in Britain are either banned or restricted in other countries. It should be remembered also that not all additives are tested for safety; the largest group, the flavourings, are not regulated at all. Not even the Ministry of Agriculture, Fisheries and Food knows which flavourings are in use in the UK and therefore they have no knowledge at all on their safety. Millstone estimates that 3,500 different flavourings are used in UK foods.

Consumer interests

Consumers are given too little information about foods. This makes it difficult to make informed, let alone healthy, decisions about which foods to eat. Although the ingredients-listing on foods provides certain details, it is inadequate. Information on the safety of any additive is deemed a commercial secret, as is the list of flavourings used. Even important details like the quantities of fat or sugar do not have to be listed and manufacturers are under no obligation to give figures. There is a good case for this information being available as a consumer's right.

The Ministry of Agriculture, Fisheries and Food launched a set of voluntary guidelines for nutritional labelling in 1987. Apart from the fact that they remain voluntary, the guidelines allow a manufacturer to provide an approved nutritional label which omits any mention of sugars, salt, dietary fibre, vitamins and minerals. This can mean that consumers buying foods like confectionery, sugar-added breakfast cereals and baked beans can be deceived as to their nutritional content. In 1979, the Food Standards Committee's Second Report on Food Labelling recommended that all future labelling legislation should be based on new principles which included:

(b) food should be sold without deceit as to its composition and character and should be so labelled as to enable a prospective purchaser to make a fair and informed choice based on clear and informed labelling.

The last principle was that '*the interests of consumers should be paramount*' (my italics).

Conclusions

The examples given show that at all stages in our food system there are avoidable risks to our health. They are not necessarily the most serious threats and are certainly not exhaustive. The important questions are: 'How can it be that the ministry which is responsible for ensuring a "safe and wholesome" food supply, has allowed these risks to persist?' and 'What, if anything, can be done now to reduce or remove such risks?'. Detailed answers are beyond the space available but we can identify the way forward.

Of course farmers and manufacturers are neither wickedly nor deliberately putting our health at risk. It is only recently that the dietary threats to health were understood sufficiently to result in a change in government policies. Even now the scope and significance of dietary risks are not universally accepted. Notice how the medical profession in Britain lags far behind their colleagues in North America in providing clear and practical advice to the public. Farmers have followed strong, if not always consistent, economic signals from the Ministry of Agriculture. During the 1970s there was a clear UK policy to expand all of its agriculture, without any real thought to the possible need to alter either the mix or the composition of products. This led to yet more milk, sugar and over-fat carcasses. The EEC is only beginning to make structural changes to agriculture and, though economics rather than health motivates the changes, they are bringing health benefits. Changing agriculture is slow and pressure should be on the policy-makers not the farmers, who are generally sympathetic, especially if they get long-term market signals they can use in planning the change.

Food manufacturers have not received the same form of support as agriculture, and the ministry has inadvertently allowed the developing industry to be established without health being a general objective of regulations. The ministry has consistently seen food safety more in terms of protecting customers from toxins or infections and stopping frauds. Indeed the origins of the present safety machinery are in the legislation dating from the end of the eighteenth century which aimed to stop bread and other foods being adulterated and short measures being served. Consumers have so far been under-represented on ministry committees like the Food Advisory Committee, which advises the minister on changes to labelling, permitted additives, novel foods etc. Since the industry has developed technologies and products for so long without health criteria being seen to be as important as hygiene, it is not surprising that so many products are now being criticised on health grounds. It is also not surprising that sectors of the food industry, especially large and powerful generic groups like dairy, sugar and red meat, are strongly resisting change. Like farmers, the manufacturers need time to make changes that the consumers and health professionals are demanding. But changes can be made.

The minister has sufficient powers under existing legislation for risks to health from food to be minimised, whether they are from permitted pesticides, the composition of milk, additives allowed in baby foods, or nutritional labelling. Clearly the first step is to give health a higher profile in food policy. The new Food Safety Act brings together much of the scattered food legislation and gives ministers wider powers should they choose to take the necessary steps. Health objectives need to be formulated and the impact of including these new health objectives in all areas of food policy needs to be examined and policies and regulations adjusted accordingly. The need for such change is evident, the means to make them are available. The missing factor is political will, but even that is emerging as consumers are becoming better informed about food than ever before and better able to press for their interests to be accommodated alongside those of the farmers and manufacturers.

REFERENCES

J. Cannon, *The Politics of Food* (London, 1987).
DHSS, *Eating for Health* (London, 1978).
House of Commons, *Effects of Pesticides on Human Health. Second Special Report of the Agricultural Committee, Session 1986-87* (London, 1987).
E. Millstone, *Food Additives: Taking the Lid Off What We Really Eat* (London, 1986).
F.W. Pavy, *A Treatise on Food and Dietetics* (London, 1874).
C.J. Robbins (ed.), *Food, Health, and Farming: Reports of Panels on the Implications for UK Agriculture* (Reading, Centre for Agricultural Strategy, 1978).
C.J. Robbins and J. Bowman, 'Nutrition and Agricultural Policy in the United Kingdom', in D.S. McLaren (ed.), *Nutrition in the Community* (Chichester, 1983).

FURTHER READING

R. Body, *Agriculture: The Triumph and the Shame* (London, 1982). A controversial but probing account of the way an effective farm lobby managed to secrete millions of pounds from the UK taxpayer with little, or at best questionable, accountability or benefit to the population.
E. Goldsmith and N. Hildyard, *Green Britain or Industrial Wasteland?* (London, 1986). A collection of essays on major environmental issues written by leading activists and experienced authors who know their subject and present an informative and compelling case for action.
P. Hausman, *Jack Sprat's Legacy. The Science and Politics of Fat & Cholesterol* (New York, 1980). An excellent account of the interaction of industry, academics and the state in resisting urgently required changes to the US daily intake of saturated fats once the links between diet and heart disease were understood from the late 1960s.
E. Morse, J. Rivers and A. Heughan, *The Family Guide to Food and Health* (London, 1988). A good mixture of practical advice on nutrition, diets, and the effects of the food and agricultural industries on food quality and composition.

Workplace transformations

Jenny Lisle

New patterns, risks and stresses

The conditions under which people work and the materials that are handled at work influence health in major ways. Work environments and work practices are changing rapidly as a result of huge technological developments in the past twenty years which are having widespread effects on industry and all types of work. The scale of the changes occurring at work today parallels the scale of Britain's industrial revolution and the rate of change outstrips anything previously seen. 'New technology' is radically altering long-established work practices and is having an ever-increasing impact on all organisations and those who work in them. The new technologies not only displace workers, but tend to reduce the classes of jobs to only two. These are:

1. Elite jobs filled only by those who know how to programme and manage technologies.
2. Service and maintenance jobs which are as poorly paid and little valued as they have always been, and some of which may be altogether displaced by new technology such as the use of robots.

Information technology, communication technology and biotechnology are among the leading technologies that will make life and work different by the twenty-first century.

New trends in work patterns are emerging, for example 'high velocity job change', especially at executive level. Short-term tenure is becoming the norm at all levels in organisations; employees are less and less likely to continue to work for the same employer for a substantial part of their working life, as their fathers and grandfathers may have done. Competitiveness is increasing, as is the pace of work. In addition workers have to live with the threat of job insecurity and redundancy. There has been a noticeable shift from manufacturing, once predominant, to service industries. Change of any kind is difficult to manage and when it is of the magnitude occurring today it has the most far-reaching consequences. All workers feel its impact, which manifests itself as stress within the organisation with consequent effects on the individual. Today's work environments contain many new hazards, often not immediately obvious but insidious and potentially damaging to health.

The Health and Safety At Work Act 1974 is the most important recent legislation concerned with occupational health and is more comprehensive than anything that preceded it, such as the Factories Act 1961. Set against a background of rising work-related accidents, the 1974 Act placed a statutory obligation upon *all* employers to secure the health, safety and welfare at work of *all* employees as far as reasonably possible, with the sole exception of domestic servants in private households. In addition the Act placed for the first time a statutory duty upon employees to take reasonable care for their own health and safety and that of their co-workers who might be affected by their acts of omission at work. The employer is required to provide and maintain a safe work environment and safe systems of work which do not endanger health. He must also provide supervision and training for employees. Anyone employing more than five persons must have a written health and safety policy. Employers also have a duty to persons other than employees and they must carry on their business in such a manner as to ensure no one outside the workplace is harmed by what goes on inside it.

The Reporting of Injuries, Diseases and Dangerous Occurrences Regulations (RIDDOR) came into force in 1986 and these require the immediate notification to the enforcing authority of serious events arising out of or in connection with work. Work can damage health in a number of ways, which may be categorised broadly as industrial accidents, specific occupational diseases and the effects of working conditions on general health (Health and Safety Executive, 1985).

The Control of Substances Hazardous to Health (COSHH) Regulations 1988 are a new piece of legislation that requires employers using materials thought to be potentially dangerous to have a health and safety audit carried out by a competent authority (Health and Safety Executive, 1988). It is very probable that more codes of practice will be established in years to come through EC influence. For example, codes similar to those already in force to control the use of lead are likely to be introduced for cadmium and mercury and probably for many of the industrial solvents.

The danger that workers will continue to be bombarded with toxic chemicals, particularly new chemicals whose effects are not immediately obvious, remains enormous, however. Electronic and other high-tech manufacturing operations involve a host of toxic substances and there is clearly a need to monitor workers' health closely in both the short and the long term. It will be necessary to take account of presumed behavioural, reproductive and carcinogenic effects and introduce measures such as genetic testing to protect susceptible workers from hazardous substances.

The National Institute for Occupational Safety and Health is part of the Center for Disease Control of the US Public Health Service. In investigating

Table 3.2   The Ten Leading Work-Related Diseases and Injuries, United States* (National Institute for Occupational Safety and Health, 1983)

1. Occupational lung diseases: asbestosis, byssinosis, silicosis, coal workers' pneumoconiosis, lung cancer, occupational asthma.

2. Musculoskeletal injuries: disorders of the back, trunk, upper extremity, neck, lower extremity; traumatically induced Raynaud's phemonenon.

3. Occupational cancers (other than lung): leukemia; mesothelioma; cancers of the bladder, nose, and liver.

4. Amputations, fractures, eye loss, lacerations, and traumatic deaths.

5. Cardiovascular diseases: hypertension, coronary artery disease, acute myocardial infarction.

6. Disorders of reproduction: infertility, spontaneous abortion, teratogenesis.

7. Neurotoxic disorders: peripheral neuropathy, toxic encephalitis, psychoses, extreme personality changes (exposure-related).

8. Noise-induced loss of hearing.

9. Dermatologic conditions: dermatoses, burns (scaldings), chemical burns, contusions (abrasions).

10. Psychologic disorders: neuroses, personality disorders, alcoholism, drug dependency.

*The conditions listed under each category are to be viewed as *selected examples*, not comprehensive definitions of the category.

health and safety hazards and workplace illness in all kinds of work environments it has developed the list of ten leading work-related diseases and injuries shown in Table 3.2.

Occupational health

There is no statutory regulation in Britain regarding any occupational health service, other than first aid, to be provided in-house for the workforce. The Health and Safety First Aid Regulations 1981, together with the accompanying approved code of practice, require an employer to provide first aid arrangements and inform all employees of such arrangements (Health and Safety Executive, 1981). Occupational health care has so far been very patchy and although some large firms have very good occupational health services the majority of small workforces (less than 250 employees) have no occupational health input. Indeed employees of many large firms also have no access to occupational health care. The Employment Medical Advisory Service set up by the Health and Safety Executive to advise employers, trade unions and others concerned with occupational health and safety, suffers from understaffing and limited resources. In 1988 the government was still considering whether to ratify the recommendations of the International Labour Organisation (ILO) that occupational health services should be extended to cover all people at work. The possibility was that the decision might be delayed for some time in view of the uncertainties about how services, particularly for small industries, should be provided and funded. People professionally concerned with occupational health are in no doubt that the recommendations ought to be followed but there is no consensus about how this can be best achieved.

So far occupational health care has grown haphazardly as a result of private initiatives, mainly by large organisations. The NHS has only recently started to develop an occupational health service for its own employees and in the financial and political climate of the late 1980s an extension to industry as a whole seems highly unlikely.

The main objectives of an occupational health service according to the definition produced by the Joint ILO/WHO Committee are:

1. to promote, maintain and improve the physical and mental well-being of workers in all occupations;
2. to advise both staff and management on the protection of employees against any physical or environmental health hazard that may arise from their work or from the conditions in which it is carried out;
3. to contribute towards workers' physical and mental adjustment to their jobs, in particular by adapting the work to the employees and by advice on the jobs for which individuals are best suited;
4. to co-ordinate occupational health functions with other health and social services.

Thus occupational health should be an important part of the health care system. Workplace medical services, however, have so far done little, with very few exceptions, to present themselves as an integral part of the health care system (House of Lords). Yet there are areas in which occupational health services could make an important contribution, for example in health promotion, the prevention of accidents and the reduction of stress-related illness.

Occupational stress

There is increasing evidence that an unsatisfactory work environment may lead to psychological disorders. Studies have shown that contributory factors are work overload, lack of control over one's work, limited job opportunities, role ambiguity and conflict, non-supportive supervisors or co-workers, and machine-paced work. Such factors create an unhealthy psychological work environment and have been linked to chronic 'stress' disorders (Fig. 3.1). Failure of top management to attend to these organisational stressors may undercut any well-intended efforts, aimed at the individual, to reduce stress through health promotion programmes. The

Figure 3.1   A model of stress at work

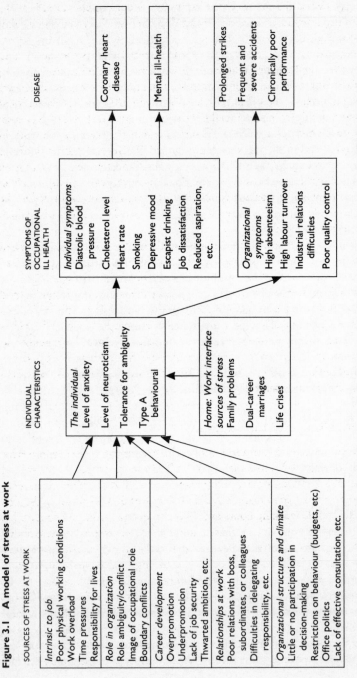

SOURCES OF STRESS AT WORK

Intrinsic to job
Poor physical working conditions
Work overload
Time pressures
Responsibility for lives

Role in organization
Role ambiguity/conflict
Image of occupational role
Boundary conflicts

Career development
Overpromotion
Underpromotion
Lack of job security
Thwarted ambition, etc.

Relationships at work
Poor relations with boss,
subordinates, or colleagues
Difficulties in delegating
responsibility, etc.

Organizational structure and climate
Little or no participation in
decision-making
Restrictions on behaviour (budgets, etc)
Office politics
Lack of effective consultation, etc.

INDIVIDUAL
CHARACTERISTICS

The individual
Level of anxiety
Level of neuroticism
Tolerance for ambiguity
Type A
behavioural

*Home: Work interface
sources of stress*
Family problems
Dual-career
marriages
Life crises

SYMPTOMS OF
OCCUPATIONAL
ILL HEALTH

Individual symptoms
Diastolic blood
pressure
Cholesterol level
Heart rate
Smoking
Depressive mood
Escapist drinking
Job dissatisfaction
Reduced aspiration,
etc.

*Organizational
symptoms*
High absenteeism
High labour turnover
Industrial relations
difficulties
Poor quality control

DISEASE

Coronary heart
disease

Mental ill-health

Prolonged strikes

Frequent and
severe accidents

Chronically poor
performance

Source: C. L. Cooper, 'Job Distress: Recent Research and the Emerging Role of the Clinical Occupational Psychologist', *Bulletin of the British Psychological Society*, 39 (1986), p. 326.

value of such programmes in the workplace would be enhanced if at the same time attention was given to tackling the organisational factors that cause stress.

Adaptation to new work practices is essential if British industry is to thrive. With enlightened management workers can adapt to new ways of working with emphasis on greater involvement and better communication throughout the organisation. This has already been demonstrated in the car industry, despite scepticism on the shopfloor about the effects of Japanese-style work practices. The Nissan plant in Sunderland is a prime example. In the United States the experiences of the laid-off General Motors workers who were re-employed at the Toyota-run plant at Freemount in California show that, with good management, the new work practices can result in considerably better working conditions. The workers all responded to the greater involvement they experienced and the increased respect with which management treated them.

Much has been said about executive stress and the pressures on people in top jobs, but there is increasing evidence that stress is experienced at all levels of organisation and can affect workers at the lowest levels more commonly since they have less control over their work environment and little scope for changing it. 'Sick Building Syndrome' may be not so much a result of physical stressors in the work environment, as a result of psycho-social stressors resulting from loss of the 'locus of control', the worker no longer having the freedom to regulate his physical environment by adjusting the lighting, heating, ventilation and so on in a modern building where the environment is centrally controlled.

Recent changes in the workforce

Employment growth in Britain has been concentrated in the service sector which now employs more than two thirds of the workforce. In the year to March 1987, service sector employment rose by 341,000, while the number of people employed in manufacturing fell by 130,000. Workplace changes include flexible working hours and increases in work done at home and in the number of part-time workers. 'Outworker sweatshops' are a growing trend. The labour market shows a noticeable shift away from full-time male work toward female part-time work. Although part-time workers now make up nearly a quarter of the working population, their role in the workplace is restricted to second-class status: they are often excluded from employers' pension and sick pay schemes and are rarely eligible to claim social security benefits.

An increase of approximately two million in the workforce over the last two decades is entirely due to the growth in the number of women working.

This means that there are now more women who combine rearing a family with a paid job and are consequently exposed to greater stress. Female patterns of morbidity and mortality are becoming more similar to male patterns.

The effects of the economic recession of the early 1980s, vast technological developments and greater international competition have been the driving forces for the changes in working practices. The growing use of new technologies in all types of industry and commerce means that the demarcation lines between manual, clerical and technical workers are fast disappearing. More people work flexi-time or part-time and companies are increasingly turning to contract or temporary staff rather than hiring full-time employees.

The huge changes in work environments and in work practices which have occurred have major implications for the health and safety of the workforces. Recommendations about occupational health and safety at work are discussed in Chapter 11.

REFERENCES

Health and Safety Executive, *Control of Substances Hazardous to Health (COSHH)* (London, 1988).

Health and Safety Executive, *First Aid Regulations* (London, 1981).

Health and Safety Executive, *A Guide to the Reporting of Injuries, Diseases and Dangerous Occurrences Regulations (RIDDOR)* (London, 1985).

House of Lords Select Committee on Science and Technology, *Occupational Health and Hygiene Services* (London, 1983).

International Labour Organisation, *Convention 161 and Recommendation 171 on Occupational Health Services* (Geneva, 1986).

National Institute for Occupational Safety and Health, 'Leading Work-Related Diseases and Injuries – United States', *Morbidity and Mortality Weekly Report*, 21 January 1983.

FURTHER READING

C. Bezold, R.J. Carlson and J.C. Peek, *The Future of Work and Health* (Dover, Mass., 1986). Provides insight into, and understanding of, the trends that affect the interplay of work and health.

R.H. Elling, *The Struggle for Workers Health: A Study of Six Industrialised Countries* (New York, 1986). A description of the widely differing arrangements for occupational health and safety in six countries (UK, Sweden, Finland, East Germany, West Germany and US).

P. Warr, *Work, Unemployment and Mental Health* (Oxford, 1987). Tackles the broad conceptual issues concerned with the effects of employment and unemployment on mental health and provides a basis for action. It recommends that all jobs should be examined for their probable impact on employee mental health and approaches to measuring mental health are considered. The book brings together factual and theoretical information in the hope that the material will suggest ways in which work environments can be designed to enhance mental health. It is suggested that work with computer-based equipment deserves particularly close scrutiny.

Unemployment, stress and health

Steve Watkins

Unemployment and ill-health

The fact that unemployment often damages the health of the families affected is not surprising. It would be expected from the fact that unemployment creates poverty, which is known to cause ill-health; affects important elements of personal psychology, like personal identity and time-structuring and self-esteem and thereby causes stress. It also adversely affects social support, which has been shown to be important to health in numerous ways. There is debate, however, as to how far unemployment affects health by means of poverty and how far it does so by means of psychological and social factors. Also, the correlations that have been found between unemployment rates and death rates in time trends, in geographical areas large and small, are open to alternative explanations.

In time trend studies, such as the much publicised and much criticised work (1971-77) of Harvey Brenner, unemployment rates are a good indicator of recession, so a correlation between unemployment rates and rates of ill-health in time trends could merely mean that recessions damage health, perhaps through their effects on working conditions, on the quality of public services, or on general levels of stress in society.

In geographical studies unemployment rates are a good indicator of multiple deprivation. Studies in various towns, from Plymouth to Newcastle, have shown that areas of the town with high unemployment rates have high death rates and sickness rates, but this could merely be documenting the effects of deprivation rather than of unemployment *per se*.

The health of unemployed people is worse than that of people in work, but this could be accounted for by health selection for unemployment/re-employment or by the fact that unemployment falls disproportionately on various unhealthy groups, e.g. low social classes, workers in declining industries, people living in areas with multiple deprivation. However, a few studies, like the British Regional Heart Survey (Cook et al), have meticulously standardised for these intervening factors and still shown the relationship between unemployment and ill-health. Such standardisation, however, is difficult and never perfect. Therefore the most relevant studies are those that follow the health of a cohort of people and take account of the various confounding factors. Such studies have confirmed that unemployment is damaging to health. A number of studies of factory closures have been done since the early work by Kasl and Cobb and most of these have confirmed their findings that the health of workers deteriorates from the time the closure first begins to be considered likely until the time the workers find alternative jobs and settle into them. A few of these studies have found the reverse, however; these have been studies into the closure of factories where working conditions have been particularly poor, showing that some work can be even more health-damaging than unemployment (Olsen and Sabroe; Westin and Norun).

The factory closure studies have been reinforced by studies that have followed the health of a cohort randomly drawn from the general population. One of the best of these was the study by Stafford, Jackson and Banks, which followed the employment experiences and mental health of a group of Leeds school-leavers from a time before they left school and before they knew whether they would get a job. Those who became unemployed had worse mental health than those who found jobs, and as there was no difference between the two groups while at school, this showed that poor mental health was not the reason for the unemployment but rather was caused by it. A much larger cohort study was the Office of Population Censuses and Surveys Longitudinal Study, which also showed that unemployment is associated with worsening health (Fox and Goldblatt; Moser et al).

Accordingly it is no longer reasonable to base policy upon any proposition other than that unemployment damages health, and this view has now even been officially acknowledged in the UK.

Psychological factors and social support

Regarding the psychological effects of unemployment, there can be no doubt that these are important, since it has been shown that the damage can be reduced by some psychological factors. These include experiences of time structuring in one's old job, low work commitment, or an attitude of mind which combines a commitment to the idea that the world can be collectively improved with a fatalistic acceptance of the personal effects of that process. However, poverty probably plays a part as well – a study on deprived estates in Oldham showed that the unemployed were unable to afford healthy diets or proper social lives (Briggs et al).

There is growing evidence of the importance to health of psychological factors. Doctors and nurses have always known that some patients will survive against the odds because they are determined to do so, whereas others will die apparently because they lack the will to live. People in general know that their health deteriorates in times of stress. It is only some people with more scientific qualifications who shied away from this folk-knowledge – and now claim to have rediscovered it.

It is well-established that working under pressure to deadlines is a risk factor for coronary heart disease; also that health deteriorates after a major life change until the individual readjusts to the changed situation. For example death rates double in the six months after bereavement. There is powerful epidemiological evidence that the strength of social support networks is a major factor in both physical and mental health. A cross-sectional epidemiological study of residents in Alameda County, California, has shown that mortality increases when the strength of social networks is reduced (Berkman and Syme). Strength of social support networks has been shown to reduce the incidence of complications of pregnancy. In the follow-up of survivors of the Granville train disaster in Australia psychiatric reactions to the horrifying experiences of the disaster were greater in those who had comparatively little social support (Boman).

The protective role of personal autonomy

Evidence is emerging that personal autonomy – control over one's life – is an important protector against stress. A recent study (Alfredson et al) has shown that the need for punctuality and low influence on choice of holidays, workmates, working hours, planning, breaks and choice of boss are all associated with raised rates of coronary heart disease and alcoholism. The biologically plausible link between psychological factors and physical ill-health is the stress reaction. This is the 'fight or flight' response which puts the body into a higher gear to cope with a threat. It is evoked whenever a human being faces a threat to its well-being, either at the level of material needs, such as warmth, shelter or financial security, or at the level of higher needs such as self-esteem, comradeship and love, personal development or opportunities to enjoy beautiful surroundings.

'Using up the stress reaction'

The stress reaction is not unhealthy in a normal situation, where it is short-lived and used up in action to counter the threat that a person faces. It becomes damaging to health when it persists. This occurs when a threat remains hanging over a person and there is nothing that he or she can do to deal with it. This is why personal autonomy is a beneficial factor; it increases the likelihood that the person will be able to use up the stress reaction in action directed at countering the threat, rather than allowing it to persist. Anyone can notice this 'using up the stress reaction' in the way the physical correlates of worry disappear, and you feel better, when you resolve upon a course of action to deal with the cause of your worry.

Conclusion

If personal autonomy is a beneficial factor in stress, as would be suggested by this theoretical approach which is borne out by some empirical evidence, this is an epidemiological argument in favour of the democratisation of society, not just in a formal representative way, but on the basis of genuine grassroots structures through which people may influence the organisations that shape their lives.

Stress affects different groups of people. It affects those who find that important elements of their destiny are taken out of their control and decided on by remote and private bureaucracies or callous governments. It also affects those who live or work in circumstances that deny their material needs, or their higher needs, and who see little prospect of escape, and therefore the poor, the unemployed and those who work involuntarily in poor conditions.

REFERENCES

L. Alfredson, C.L. Spetz and J. Theorell, 'Type of Occupation and Near Future Hospitalisation for Myocardial Infarction and some other Diagnoses', *International Journal of Epidemiology*, 14, 3 (1985).

L.F. Berkman and S.L. Syme, 'Social Networks, Host Resistance and Mortality: A Nine Year Follow Up of Alameda County Residents', *American Journal of Epidemiology*, 109 (1979).

B. Boman, 'Behavioural Observations on the Granville Train Disaster and the Significance of Stress for Psychiatry', *Social Sciences and Medicine*, 13A (1979).

M.H. Brenner, 'Economic Changes and Heart Disease Mortality', *American Journal of Public Health*, 61, 3 (1971).

M.H. Brenner, 'Foetal, Infant and Maternity Mortality During Periods of Economic Instability', *International Journal of Health Services*, 3, 2 (1973).

M.H. Brenner, 'Health Costs and Benefits of Economic Policy', *International Journal of Health Services*, 7, 4 (1977).

M.H. Brenner, *Mental Illness and the Economy* (Cambridge, Mass., 1973).

Briggs et al, *The Effects of the Recession on the Lives and Health of the People in Two Underprivileged Areas of Oldham* (Oldham, Oldham Resources and Information Centre, 1987).

S.M. Cobb, G.W. Brooks, S.V. Kasl and W.E. Connelly, 'The Health of People Changing Jobs: a Description of a Longitudinal Study', *American Journal of Public Health*, 156, 9 (1966).

D.G. Cook, R.O. Cummins, M.J. Bartley and A.G. Shaper, 'Health of Unemployed Middle Aged Men in Great Britain', *The Lancet*, 5 June 1982.

A.J. Fox and R.O. Goldblatt, *Longitudinal Study: Socio-Demographic Mortality Differentials 1971-75*, Series LS No. 1 (London, 1982).

L. Iversen and H. Glausen, 'Lukringen af Nardhavn – Vaerflet', *Institute for Social Medicine*, Publication 13 (University of Copenhagen, 1981).

S.V. Kasl and S.M. Cobb, 'Blood Pressure Changes in Men Undergoing Job Loss: A Preliminary Report', *Psychosomatic Medicine*, 32, 1 (1970).

K.A. Moser, A.J. Fox, D.R. Jones and P.O. Goldblatt, 'Unemployment and Mortality: Further Evidence from the OPCS Longitudinal Study 1971-81', *The Lancet*, 15 February 1986.

J. Olsen and S. Sabroe, 'A Follow-Up Study of Non-Retired Members of the Danish Carpenter/Cabinet Makers' Trade Union', *International Journal of Epidemiology*, 8, 4 (1979).

E.M. Stafford, P.R. Jackson and M.H. Banks, 'Employment, Work Involvement and Mental Health in Less Qualified Young People', *Journal of Occupational Psychology*, 53 (1980).

S. Westin and D. Norun, *Naar Sardinfabrikken Nedlegges* (Bergen, Norway, Institut for Hygiene og Sosialmedesin, 1977).

Only the major references have been given. Where statements in the text are not supported by references support will be found in the literature review by the Unemployment and Health Study Group, listed in Further Reading.

FURTHER READING

Unemployment and Health Study Group, *Unemployment: A Challenge to Public Health*, Occasional Paper No. 10 (University of Manchester: Centre for Professional Development, Department of Community Medicine, 1984). This is a thorough literature review of the subject, which has been used as the base for the discussion in this chapter and which also contains a report of a conference on policy implications of unemployment and health.

R. Smith, *Unemployment and Health* (Oxford, 1987). Another comprehensive review of the subject, based on a series of articles in the British Medical Journal.

J. John, D. Schwefel and H. Zollner, 'Influence of Economic Instability on Health', *Lecture Notes on Medical Informatics*, 21 (Berlin, 1983).

G. Westcott, P.G. Svensson and H.F.K. Zollner, *Health Policy Implications of Unemployment* (Copenhagen, WHO Regional Office for Europe, 1985).

Papers of the 1987 Conference on Unemployment, Poverty and the Quality of Working Life (Vienna, European Centre for Social Welfare Training and Research, 1987). Also forthcoming soon in book form. These are the papers of a series of conferences organised by the WHO Regional Office for Europe on the subject of unemployment and health. They contain a fascinating combination of empirical research, review articles and research proposals which paint a vivid picture of debate and the development of understanding. These comprehensive publications cover the two Munich conferences and the Vienna conference. Reports of the Copenhagen and Ljubljana conferences are also available but are more selective.

Parenting and public health
Jo Tunnard

The links between parenting and public health may be considered from various angles. One is to reflect on personal experiences, teasing out the factors that seem to have made for a positive sense of well-being and confidence during spells of parenting. Another is to draw together the research studies that have examined, for instance, the mental health of young mothers, parents' access to job opportunities and good-quality daycare provision, or the experiences of parents left alone again after children have grown up. I want to tackle the issue from a rather different angle: to consider the experiences of those parents who turn, or are turned, to statutory agencies in times of difficulty and who, by so doing, may find that their role as parents is placed in jeopardy. There is much to be learnt from the experiences of those parents about the pressures of child rearing, the aspirations of parents for themselves and for their children, and the sort of response that they expect the state to provide. My comments are drawn from the experiences of the Family Rights Group over the past ten years of advising families with children in public care and of advising and training professional workers and others about child care law and good practice.

The families who end up with their children in care are no different from many other families, including our own, who struggle along together. It is our experience that most parents who have been separated from their children – voluntarily or under compulsion by a local authority – are hard-pressed but caring people who desperately want to provide for their own children but lack the resources to do so. Many of the families whom we have advised have been denied, or have had limited, access to the kind of facilities that would be a help to parents looking after their children – gardens, play spaces, nurseries, playgroups. When these facilities are not available the stresses and strains of child care are made more acute when families feel trapped by having to live in high-rise flats or small, cramped rooms on stigmatised and vandalised estates. In addition to these physical constraints the poverty they experience burdens them with the added pressures of threatened or actual fuel disconnection, of queuing for hours for benefit giros that have been delayed or lost in the post, or struggling with bills for food, rent and clothing that can never all be paid in full.

Poverty

While some children are removed from their parents for reasons in no way connected with poverty, considerable evidence points to a relationship between social deprivation and the taking of children into public care. One strong indicator is that children admitted to care come disproportionately from depressed urban areas or those parts of local authorities that are characterised by extensive poverty, overcrowding and inadequate housing conditions. Another indicator is the family income of those involved in the care system. Official statistics make no provision for recording a child's entry on account of poverty, but numerous small-scale research studies show that most children in care are from families at or below the state poverty level at the time of family separation.

Poverty promotes three further deprivations that can impair family behaviour. First, the poor are more liable to physical ill-health which, in turn, can seriously impair parenting capacities. Second, the poor may be denied the prerequisites for a normal development of a child's social skills. Third, parents may be deprived of self-respect and positive self-image. In our society, such feelings depend on being able to participate, on being able to contribute as well as to take. Unable to provide, unable to participate in normal life, perhaps handicapped by ill-health, poor parents are made to feel inferior as they fail to provide for the needs of their children and fail to get the resources that they believe will help them provide well for their families.

Daycare

The unmet demand for daycare places remains staggeringly high. One result is that families who cannot afford to pay for daycare themselves and so turn to the local authority for help, may find that there is no provision available or no choice about the sort of service that suits them best. To gain access to those services that they cannot afford some families have to demonstrate that they have already failed their children; in many areas a daycare place is granted only after it is thought that the child has suffered non-accidental injury. In other areas parents who do not have paid work are not considered to be in need of a daycare place. It is policy in some local authorities to use sponsored child-minders rather than offering the choice of nursery, playgroup, child-minder or family centre. One mother who recently contacted the Family Rights Group had been refused a daycare place for her toddler because her social worker considered that the mother did not have a good enough relationship with her son to merit their having a place.

It is our view that parents generally know what is best for themselves and their children and that they want daycare provision because they know it benefits both them and their children. Rather than targeting provision on those deemed to be in need, as happens in many areas, or leaving the amount of provision to the discretion of the local authority, we believe that there should be legislation to underpin the general principle that facilities should be available for all children and all families.

Housing

A family's cramped, unhealthy or otherwise inadequate housing can have long-term effects on all involved. Some eight years ago the National Children's Bureau defined disadvantaged children as those from a family of four or more children or with only one parent, living on a low income, and growing up in poor housing conditions. The overall effect of these three factors is children 'born to fail'. The under-achievement that consistently occurs under such conditions can not be attributed to something inside the children, but is due to the circumstances of their life. And the Select Committee on Violence in the Family – while stressing that non-accidental injury occurs in all social classes – has pointed to the tensions created by poor housing conditions:

> We were impressed by the number of parents we saw who had experienced severe housing problems which contributed to their difficulties with their children . . . inadequate housing produces a great deal of stress in parents and can turn difficult but normal circumstances of child upbringing into almost impossible ones. A crying, teething baby needs a lot of patience even in adequate housing, but where a family is sharing accommodation or in a bedsitter, or in badly sound-proofed accommodation, the worry of the crying upsetting other people can create very great strain. Similarly, trying to keep quiet or keep others quiet so that a baby can sleep, produces great strain in cramped conditions.

The Housing (Homeless Persons) Act 1977 did much to reduce the number of separated families by placing a duty on local authorities to house children with their parents. But there are still 100,000 families classified as homeless and the quality of housing remains to be tackled. The current restrictions on housing expenditure will increase the plight of many families who are waiting for improvements and repairs to be done or who are desperate for a decent home of their own. We should not underestimate the extent to which appalling living conditions can push the stress level in families just that much too far for otherwise capable people.

We should not underestimate, either, the stresses caused to parents and children when state intervention does not resolve their housing problems. The most recent government statistics for England and Wales reveal that 8,402 children are separated from their parents and living in public care because of homelessness or unsatisfactory housing conditions. Three of our Group's most difficult cases involve families who, at the birth of their child, had nowhere decent to live. Two families were in caravans, one with a leaking roof and the other exceptionally draughty. The third mother was deserted by her husband a week before her child's birth, went to her parents' home until friction caused her to leave, and subsequently had to leave a mother-and-baby home with her baby when she objected to the matron's proposal to place two more babies and their mothers in her small room. In all three cases the social services department was alerted to the inadequate housing conditions and the children were received into or committed to care and placed with foster carers. In all three cases, and while the housing problems persisted, the parents were told that they might never see their children again. One of the children has already been adopted against the wishes of his parents.

Public care

If children are admitted to care we have found that parents experience very similar reactions. They often feel that losing a child to public care is the most devastating thing that can happen to them. They feel they have failed their children and they believe that their neighbours, friends, family and social workers see them as failures too. They tend to shrink away from contact with their friends and they get visited less frequently than before by their social workers. They often find they are just as busy as when they had their children with them, because of meetings with social services, solicitors, social security officers and court officials. They find that the welfare benefits that caused them worries before now seem to get hopelessly muddled. Some parents find that, having responded to the suggestion that their children go into care, the next thing that happens is that they get a demand for payment to the local authority toward the cost of their child's keep.

Visiting their children can be a further blow to their self-esteem. It is not unusual for parents to end up feeling that there is nothing they can do but sit back and watch their children being well cared for by strangers. They lose their role as parents, feel distraught at seeing their children in surroundings that they would want to be able to provide, and are just as upset when their children cry when they leave them. Arranging visits can create added stress, especially if children are placed a long distance from their family.

A mother's social worker said that she had unrestricted access to her five year old daughter in care. In order to use the 'unrestricted access' the mother, who lived 100 miles from the office and the same distance from her daughter, had to phone the social worker from a public call box and find her in, and not in a team meeting, in supervision, seeing a client in the office or out on a visit. Having had the request for a visit, the social worker would have to speak to the foster family to find out when it would be convenient. The mother would then have to call back, and again usually several times, before getting to speak to the social worker and hearing the arrangements that had been made. The mother then travelled the 100 miles on public transport, financed it out of her supplementary benefit (income support) and waited for the money to be repaid to her later. After the visit she had to start the whole process again to set up her next 'unrestricted' access visit. All these manoeuvres meant that the mother and daughter met each other only once every three months. The social worker's view was the arrangements should be made through her; she had no concept of the hoops and hurdles involved for the mother. (Atherton).

I am not using this example to suggest that such difficulties arise out of deliberate thoughts and actions by the local authority or individual workers. What seems more probable is that most difficulties are the direct result of people not thinking hard enough about the effect of admitting children to public care and its impact on everyone's feelings. The problem does not arise only in relation to visits that parents make to their children. It can happen also when children return home to visit their parents and other relatives.

A father that we are advising is unemployed and disabled and therefore dependent on social security benefits. His middle child, a teenage boy, is in public care. He comes home every three weeks and stays from Friday to Sunday. His parents travel into central London to meet him off the train and take him back to the main-line station at the end of the weekend. Last time he was home his mother replaced some small items of clothing, and the boy went to a football match with his brother on the Saturday afternoon. Food apart, his parents spent £6 on his care. But they got no support to do that. As the boy was not at home each and every weekend his mother did not qualify for child benefit for him and his father did not qualify for a child addition to his invalidity benefit. At the end of the weekend the couple were desperate that their son should continue to join in their family life as often as possible but could not imagine how they would be able to afford to pay for their boy's next visit home. (Atherton)

Models of good practice

Fortunately, there are many examples that people can draw on to press for policies and practices that would do much to promote the health and well-being of parents and their children.

Individual work with families

Some families, once rehoused, have the time, the space and the energy to cope with other difficulties without help.

A single parent with four children aged between eight and fourteen was referred to a social work agency because it was feared that the mother would have another nervous breakdown. She had received psychiatric treatment in the past. The housing conditions were bad and the family income came from income support. The eldest girl had been cautioned for shoplifting and her mother was afraid to let her out in the evening as they lived in the city's red-light area. One of the boys banged his head against the bedroom wall at night. His violent rocking sometimes collapsed his bed and continually woke his brother and sister who shared the same room. The other boy wet the bed every night. Their mother complained about the house. The only water supply was in the kitchen and that had just a small water heater. There was no bathroom and only an outside toilet. One of the bedrooms was too damp to use and there was nowhere for the children to play or entertain their friends.

The agreed aim of social work intervention was rehousing. It took five months of negotiations with the local authority before the family was offered a modern, three-bedroomed, centrally-heated home. The daughter was allowed out at night and the mother's anxiety ceased. The youngest boy did not wet the bed again. The other boy was given a legless bed in the middle of the floor and told to rock as much as he wanted because it did not matter and would not disturb anyone. This habit simply died away.

Community social work

Workers at a new family centre were faced with the problems of how to involve parents who had been referred to the centre with their children: parents whose initial expectations were that the centre was for the children, not for them; who had been referred because they were deemed to be 'at risk'; and who saw the centre as a nursery where you left your children and went, rather than getting anything out of it for yourself by staying and joining in.

The workers began by running a discussion group each week, which included a carefully selected outside health professional who was not intimidating and had something of interest to say. Quite quickly the parents demanded their own personal discussion group and this ran side by side with the other more formal group. The recurrent theme was to do with depression and relationships. Issues debated and wrestled with were concerned with health, and included personal well-being, eating, managing ailments, and rearing children on poverty income. About a year later, and arising out of the group work, the centre set up the first of what came to be described as health days. They consisted of group discussion, talks, yoga and relaxation, and an opportunity to browse through health-related material.

Those involved in the project point to various advantages of such an approach. It gave parents skills in integrating new members into the group as well as including people who did not always fit into what is considered acceptable and normal behaviour. It gave parents who have been oppressed by health bureaucracies access to complicated information about health in an easy and palatable manner. It freed them to spend time thinking and talking about themselves, their relationships and their environment. And it gave some of the parents the confidence to try new ways of tackling long-standing health problems.

Self-help groups for parents

In 1983 the Family Rights Group, funded by grants from charitable trusts, initiated a project aimed at encouraging the formation of self-help groups for parents and other relatives of children in care. A modest independent evaluation of these groups and of the Family Rights Group's efforts was built into the project and its findings have since been published (Monaco and Thoburn). The most compelling finding was the contrast between the very positive comments about the helpfulness of the groups and the more negative view of the help received from the social services department, especially at the time when the children went into care. All the parents considered that the social workers were the children's workers and several commented on their inability to trust the social workers. Typical comments were: 'They didn't care at all about me as a person or a mother. They are totally against parents' feelings of love toward their children', and 'She said she was only acting on the children's behalf'. In contrast, self-help groups were seen as successful in a variety of ways, but especially because they offered information and support both with emotional turmoil and with negotiations with social services. The majority spoke as positively of their ability to help others in the group as of the group's role in helping them.

The research report highlights many tips for good practice for social workers and self-help group co-ordinators. In essence, the conclusion is that the choice is not 'either groups or social work'. Social workers must provide an effective service to parents as well as children, in the interest of both. But other parents who have gone through the experience themselves are in a better position to provide the whole-hearted support, advocacy and friendship that can help fight off the depression and despair of some parents, and channel the anger of others, so that children and their families benefit from improved services.

REFERENCES

C. Atherton, *Promoting Links: Keeping Children and Families in Touch* (London, Family Rights Group, 1986), Chapter 4.

M. Monaco and J. Thoburn, *Self-Help for Parents with Children in Care* (Norwich, 1987).

Select Committee on Violence in the Family, *First Report* (London, 1977), para. 80.

FURTHER READING

D.H.S.S., *Social Work Decisions in Child Care – Recent Research Findings and their Implications* (London, 1985). A useful summary of nine research studies into the circumstances of some two thousand children in care in England and Wales. It pulls out the common findings that have a bearing on professional and practice issues regarding social work decisions about children and their families and state care.

Jane Tunstill (ed.), *In Care in North Battersea* (Guildford, 1987). A study of the views of parents, children and social workers about the care system in one part of inner London. With information and discussion about the link between poverty and care, and between research and policy developments.

C. Atherton, *Promoting Links: Keeping Children and Families in Touch* (London, Family Rights Group, The Print House, 18 Ashwin Street, London E8 3DL, 1986). £4 inc. postage. A collection of papers about the difficulties that families and children experience in trying to maintain good links with each other when children are in public care.

Marianne Monaco and June Thoburn, *Self-Help for Parents with Children in Care* (Norwich, 1987). An evaluation of the use of local self-help groups for parents and other relatives of children in care, and for the social workers involved. Includes a description of the work that groups do, their successes and problems, and the questionnaire used for the study. £4 from Family Rights Group.

CHAPTER 4

Other risks and stresses of urban life

We now look at some specific and mainly new problems of twentieth-century living. We start with health problems met in tapping various energy sources – fossil fuels and nuclear, wind, water, solar and geothermal. We then explore the very direct impacts on health of town and country planning and transport, and identify changes needed to make the day-to-day physical environment less damaging.

Energy comes poisoned

Steve Watkins

Energy is important for health but its production often damages it. Therein lies the core of the problem of healthy energy policy. Energy is important for health for two main reasons. It is essential for the operation of modern industrial processes and, to the extent that those processes meet genuine human needs, it is therefore essential for the beneficial consequences of these. Secondly, energy is essential for heat, and there is a close and almost certainly causal association between cold and ischaemic heart disease.

There is no healthy way to produce energy on the scale it is currently used by industrialised countries. Coal mining has one of the highest accident rates of any occupation, as well as high mortality from respiratory diseases. Indiscriminate burning of coal, wood or oil causes air pollution, and its legacy of chronic bronchitis still burdens generations who grew up before clean air legislation. Nuclear energy seems safer, but has an inbuilt potential for disasters on a world-wide scale. Wind, tidal, solar and geothermal energy tap ecological sources that have so far produced only relatively small amounts of energy, though with outstanding safety. Some dam schemes have had ecological consequences which teach us that hydro-electric power, once seen as a clean and cheap source of energy, is not in fact free of costs to health or the environment.

Transport of energy is also hazardous. Carrying oil brings risk of explosion or spillage. Gas pipes explode. Pylons blow down, casting high-voltage electric cables loose; there is also a suggestion that these cables can damage people's health nearby through the impact of abnormal magnetic fields on the human body. Gas, electricity and fire are dangerous to use. Nor is minimising their use by energy conservation without risk: radio-activity due to radon from the natural content of brick and rock has been shown to rise in houses where heat loss is prevented. Energy is our lifeblood – but it comes with poisons. It harms us but we cannot live without it.

The effect of energy on people's health should also be seen in a context of wider peril, involving the health of generations to come and possibly human survival. Today's primary sources of energy are mainly non-renewable: natural gas, oil, coal, peat and conventional nuclear power. There are also renewable resources, including wood, plants, dung, falling water, tidal, wind and wave energy as well as human and animal muscle-power. Each energy source carries its own economic and environmental costs, benefits and risks in addition to the direct effects on personal health. A global survey, *Our Common Future*, done for the World Commission on Environment and Development, noted in its 1987 report: 'Choices must be made in the certain knowledge that choosing an energy strategy inevitably means choosing an environmental strategy . . . A generally acceptable pathway to a safe and sustainable energy future has not yet been found'.

The commission, chaired by Norwegian Prime Minister Gro Harlem Brundtland, identified the key elements of sustainability that have to be reconciled as:

* sufficient growth of energy supplies to meet human needs (which means accommodating a minimum of 3 per cent per capita income growth in developing countries);
* energy efficiency and conservation measures so that waste of primary resources is minimised;
* public health, recognising the problems of risks to safety inherent in energy sources; and
* protection of the biosphere and prevention of more localised forms of pollution. (World Commission on Environment and Development, p. 169)

Hazards

The report warns: 'We all depend on one biosphere for sustaining our lives.

Yet each community, each country, strives for survival and prosperity with little regard for its impact on others. Some consume the Earth's resources at a rate that would leave little for future generations. Others, many more in number, consume far too little and live with the prospects of hunger, squalor, disease, and early death' (p. 27). Brundtland writes in her preface:

> The present decade has been marked by a retreat from social concerns. Scientists bring to our attention urgent but complex problems bearing on our very survival: a warming globe, threats to the Earth's ozone layer, deserts consuming agricultural land . . . Environmental degradation, first seen as mainly a problem of the rich nations, and a side effect of industrial wealth, has become a survival issue for developing nations. It is part of the downward spiral of linked ecological and economic decline in which many of the poorest nations are trapped. (p. xi)

Emissions of the principal pollutants of the atmosphere were greatly reduced, mainly in cities in the most developed countries, by some of the controls introduced from the late 1960s on. Yet at the same time emissions rose to serious levels in cities in several industrial and newly industrialised countries, some of which are by now the world's most polluted urban areas (United Nations Environment Programme, p. iii). A report from the richest nations' economic organisation noted:

> Atmospheric pollution, once seen only as a local urban-industrial problem involving people's health, is now also seen as a much more complex issue encompassing buildings, ecosystems and maybe even public health over vast regions. During transport in the atmosphere, emissions of sulphur and nitrogen oxides and volatile hydrocarbons are transformed into sulphuric and nitric acids, ammonium salts, and ozone. They fall to the ground, sometimes many hundreds of thousands of miles from their origins, as dry particles or in rain, snow, frost, fog and dew. Few studies of their socio-economic costs are available, but these show that they are considerable and suggest that they are rapidly increasing. (Organisation for Economic Co-operation and Development)

The Brundtland Report notes that energy is a mix of products and services that have been allowed to flow together haphazardly. Its conclusion:

Energy is too important for its development to continue in such a random manner. A safe, environmentally sound, and economically viable energy pathway that will sustain human progress into the distant future is clearly imperative. It is also possible. But it will require new dimensions of political will and institutional co-operation to achieve it. (p. 202)

Energy and health

The wider range of the health consequences of economic activity will be examined in Chapter 9. Here we note simply that industry which is uncontrolled, has poor working conditions, and no regard for the environment or safety – as was common in the nineteenth century – damages health. In that century health actually improved during economic recessions; in this century, industry in controlled environmental and working conditions has been associated with improving health in a context of economic growth. If economic activity is today, on balance, good for health, it follows that the energy needed for that activity is a health-promoting force.

A more direct health-promoting use of energy is in heating. Cold kills people. For each 1°C fall in mean weekly temperature there were two extra deaths from ischaemic heart disease per week per million population in London, according to a study conducted in the early 1970s. It is necessary to specify date and place, because it must be supposed that atmospheric temperature affects the ambient temperature of the human body and therefore the effect of cold will be greater in areas where individuals are less well protected by heating or clothes. Poorer areas, and the poor in any area, are likely to be most affected.

This effect is not to be confused with hypothermia, which occurs only in very low temperatures and is a problem of much less numerical importance. The fact that a few old people die of hypothermia each severe winter is horrifying and attracts media attention. The fact that fit young people die of heart attacks in increased numbers when the temperature starts to fall below that of a warm spring day is a much greater public health problem that attracts much less attention (West, Lloyd and Roberts). So it is healthy to wear warm clothes and turn up the central heating as it gets cold. This healthy behavioural norm is more prevalent among the middle classes than among the poor. This is not because the middle classes are more intelligent or well-informed about the need for a warm lifestyle, it is because they can afford to turn up the heating.

Equitable distribution of life-saving energy is one of the first elements of a health-promoting energy policy. Nobody should be financially unable to keep warm, and a nation in which people shiver in cold houses or on the streets in winter for lack of money is on a par with a nation in which people starve. If it is a rich nation the existence of that state of affairs indicates that the nation lacks some essential features of common humanity; if a poor nation, it indicates that the world economic system and the nations that benefit from it lack those features. Britain, the United States and most of the countries of Western Europe stand indicted on the first count and all the countries of the developed world, without exception, stand indicted on the second. Gandhi was right when, asked what he thought of western civilisation, he replied that it would be a good idea.

The noble coughing miner

The image of women and children clustered round the pit-head waiting for news of the victim of an accident is graven on our cultural memory. The death-rate among miners is 50 per cent higher than among the general workforce. Miners suffer two-and-a-half times as much chronic bronchitis as the rest of the population, and much of the bronchitis suffered by the non-mining population is caused by the burning of coal. Industries ran on coal and smothered surrounding towns beneath a black pall of smoke. In the Pennine towns of Lancashire and Yorkshire it was impossible to see the bottom of the valleys from the tops of the surrounding hills. It is only since the Clean Air Act 1956 that the people of those valleys have seen the bright red of Accrington brick or the beautiful golden colour of the local stone buildings. Until then they had lived in the belief that all buildings were black. The local pathologists had the same delusion about lung tissue.

One idea that should be stricken from any healthy energy policy is the idea that a growing part of our energy needs should be met by a product which is won and used at such human cost. We need to confine the production of coal to those situations in which it can be relatively easily extracted without the human cost associated with so many of the more marginal pits, and we need to confine the production of energy by burning things within the limits the ecosystem can tolerate.

Fifty years ago the labour movement universally regarded it as unacceptable that noble miners coughed their way to the grave for the profits of mine owners. It is equally unacceptable that they cough their way to the grave for the sake of cheap energy for the people. Of course the closure of pits must, to be healthy, be carried through with due regard to the problems of the communities dependent on the industry. The problem is similar to problems of diversification in the tobacco or arms industries.

Nuclear energy

Nuclear energy has an enviable safety record. Although the waste
from Windscale may have caused some deaths from malignancies, this
is not out of scale with the deaths caused by other industries and
Windscale was an early plant which has been much improved on in
later designs. There have been very few accidents in the industry and
its attention to safety is a model for other industries.

So might run the nuclear industry's defence of itself and it is superficially
convincing. However, the Chernobyl disaster caused contamination across
the whole of Western Europe. It came close to destroying the entire
agricultural productive capacity of the Ukraine for a generation. America's
Three-Mile Island disaster came very close to a core meltdown that would
have released huge quantities of radioactive waste and caused thousands of
deaths. It is on this potential for a megadisaster that nuclear energy must be
assessed.

What cost do we ascribe to a very small but real danger of a disaster that
will cause thousands or even millions of deaths and destroy the ecology of a
vast area making it unproductive and uninhabitable for a long period of
time? This is the question that must be asked about the safety of the nuclear
industry; raising questions about its existing safety figures merely distracts
our attention.

The dangers do not stop at the possibility of a megadisaster. There is a
further problem. 'A' level physics, some imagination, a well-equipped
workshop, some basic craft ability, the willingness to die of radiation
sickness as a result of working without adequate safety precautions, and a
quantity of enriched plutonium are all that is necessary to build an atomic
bomb (more extensive facilities would be necessary in the absence of a
death-wish). This fact has presumably not escaped the notice of terrorist
groups. And the only one of these prerequisites that a terrorist could not
easily possess is the enriched plutonium. The nuclear industry, however,
produces the material in abundance – and terrorists need only steal it to
have the capacity to destroy cities. I do not doubt the immense security
apparatus that exists to prevent the theft of enriched plutonium, I do not
doubt the checks and double-checks on the stability and honesty of those
who operate it, the careful accountancy, the hidden checks, the strength of
the guard system, the care and ingenuity with which security alarms have
been designed. But history has shown anything can be stolen.

If the operation of an industry that has the potential for megadisaster
and produces a material that terrorists could use to destroy an entire city is
not enough evidence of irresponsibility, let us consider the third criticism of

the nuclear industry. In the hope, but by no means the certainty, that we will find a way of decontaminating nuclear waste, the industry produces material that will remain deadly for 10,000 years. If the Romans had had nuclear energy we would still be looking after their waste!

Conclusion

A healthy energy policy must reduce the use of coal and abandon the use of nuclear energy. It must replace these losses with vigorous energy conservation and the use of solar, wind, tidal and geothermal sources of energy. The energy produced must be used in a healthy pattern of economic activity and made available to maintain a human right to warmth. We must not rely so heavily on any one source of energy that we allow the dangers of that source to become critical. Once we seized greedily on the smoke-dispersing power of the high wind currents and used them so much that we overwhelmed them and it is painful for us to recreate an atmosphere that is polluted only to an acceptable degree. We must not repeat that mistake with the winds, the tides, the sun and the warmth of the earth.

We must not take the lifeblood so greedily that we fail to notice the poison in it.

REFERENCES

Organisation for Economic Co-operation and Development, *The State of the Environment* (Paris, 1985).
United Nations Environment Programme, *The State of the World Environment* (Nairobi, UNEP, 1987).
R.R. West, S. Lloyd and C.J. Roberts, 'Mortality from Ischaemic Heart Disease – Association with Weather', *British Journal of Social and Preventive Medicine*, 27, 1 (1973).
World Commission on Environment and Development, *Our Common Future* (The Brundtland Report) (New York, WCED, 1987).

FURTHER READING

WHO, *Health Impact of Different Energy Sources: A Challenge for the End of the Century* (Copenhagen, WHO Regional Office for Europe, 1986). This is a report of a study group. The group drew up a model matrix of the different kinds of health risk from each fuel cycle. The number and severity of problems of the various energy sources increases from water, gas and the sun to oil, nuclear energy and coal. The matrix is only a preliminary assessment and the group indicated remaining gaps in knowledge.

Planning and health

Reg Harman

The history of town planning in Britain, especially over the last hundred years, has generally been associated with improvements in public health. The early nineteenth century saw large numbers of people moving from agriculture into manufacturing as the industrial age burgeoned; towns grew apace, and the resultant overcrowding led to major epidemics, such as cholera. In response, philanthropy and commercial interests combined to regulate minimum design standards for streets and houses, to create a healthier environment. The early twentieth century brought the garden city movement, which promoted visionary new towns in which areas, streets and buildings were designed to create communities and households free from the urban squalor of the period.

During the first half of this century town planning developed as a legal system and a professional responsibility, primarily based on planning and control of development by local authorities. It aimed to bring a civilising influence to the form of settlements, creating a pleasant environment in which everyone could enjoy convenient and healthy lifestyles. In some respects it brought substantial achievements: cities, towns and villages have been restrained from excessive sprawl by the setting of standards for minimum open space, the establishment of green belts and similar controls.

Current town planning still shows serious weaknesses, however. The control of development by local authorities as the prime mechanism is formal and reactive and can prove inflexible. In any case, development is brought about by many factors, which the town planning system can only guide. Amid the rapid changes of recent decades the system has retained features that have become irrelevant or even anti-social. Two main ways in which this has affected health are seen in the design of settlements and buildings and in the emphasis which town planning places on the accommodation of motor traffic.

Settlement and building design

Town planning approaches settlement design on the principle of defining separate zones for particular activities. Originally there were good reasons for this, notably the aim of keeping residential areas free from the noise and pollution caused by industrial processes. Today many industrial activities cause little pollution; zoning, however, has produced in many towns residential estates that lack both facilities and employment close at hand. In consequence many people suffer damaging stress from loneliness and from difficulties in obtaining services. The 'new town blues' of the 1950s also affect today's low-density private estates (an issue explored in 'Tomorrow-land', a major ITV documentary programme in 1987). With little sense of place and community, such areas can breed vandalism and violence. Modern layouts, especially those formed of machine-built high-density housing, often include grassed areas that meet statutory requirements on open space and look pleasant on plans, but whose indefinite role and lack of 'ownership' merely add to social problems. These problems are seen at their worst in tower blocks of flats, which have become clearly associated with severe isolation and violence.

These examples of housing illustrate another problem – the failure of town planners to insist on building designs that use energy efficiently. Many dwellings in Britain are far more expensive to heat than they need be, because of poor insulation and siting. In fact, for a relatively small extra building cost it is possible to achieve massive savings in domestic consumption; in Canada and Sweden, for example, high standards of energy efficiency are the norm (Hillman and Bollard, Chapter 1). The excessive use of energy necessary simply to keep warm leads many elderly people and families either to suffer in cold and uncomfortable homes or to divert money from other necessities: either way it increases health risks. Hypothermia among elderly people during severe cold has understandably roused particular public concern in recent years.

Town planning has tended to concentrate – albeit implicitly – on providing housing that can accommodate a nuclear family. Although the number of small, fragmented families has increased considerably during the 1980s, a high proportion of new dwellings are family houses, usually three-bedroom (see for example the Annual Monitors of the London & SE Regional Planning Conference). This has restricted the extent to which property can be shared by groups or otherwise used more flexibly. It has also tied in with a continuing trend for people to own their home rather than rent it. This too can cause problems, because a private home represents a substantial personal commitment; many people now find serious financial pressures in maintaining one. If the home is uncomfortable to live in and structurally less than perfect, health and well-being can be affected, for instance by poverty and worry over fuel bills. For younger couples this may lead to delay in starting a family or excessive working hours to increase earnings: both may lead to damaging stress. Elderly home-owners can be forced to look for sheltered accommodation before they really need it; this works against the current policy of keeping elderly people in the community as long as possible, because independence tends to maintain their mental health.

Town planning and motor vehicles

Over the last forty years most development plans have given substantial priority to accommodating the use of motor vehicles in towns and cities, and this has heavily influenced urban form. Planning has concentrated on responding to these pressures, aiming to link zones by suitable roads. Rising traffic levels have been seen as evidence of need for more capacity rather than as the result of providing it. Economics and technology have also led toward larger and more remote facilities which increase the need to travel, such as hypermarkets, industrial or business 'parks' and large secondary schools. Such development is associated with the rundown of equivalent facilities in neighbourhood or town centres. Town planning has generally tried to cater for this rather than seek to contain it. This approach contrasts with the policy followed in many countries, including some that are generally looked on as liberal in attitude towards consumer possessions. For example, Gothenburg in Sweden limits town centre congestion by comprehensive traffic management; it complements this with a good passenger transit system, round which the newer suburbs are planned. The same principles, on a larger scale, are followed in Stockholm. A number of smaller Dutch and West German towns have also adopted this approach.

The need to travel further has brought two main effects. First, people's health has suffered directly from excessive and unrestrained use of motor vehicles, which is discussed in the next section. Second, by allowing settlement structure to adapt to traffic domination, town planners have reinforced the patterns of remoteness and lack of local facilities caused by the separation of activity zones. Contrary to popular belief, car ownership is far from universal. In 1985, of all households in Britain, about one-third had no car, and only one in five owned two cars or more (Department of Transport). As residential areas and public and commercial facilities become more widely separated, many people are often unable to reach even basic services except at high cost and inconvenience. This results in more stress and less personal care. Elderly and young people, as well as families in more dependent circumstances, suffer particularly: the 1985 statistics also showed that the proportion of households with no car was 44 per cent among semi-skilled households, 60 per cent among retired households, and 62 per cent among unskilled households. Local public transport (especially conventional bus services) has seen falling service levels over the last twenty years.

Substantial benefits to people's health and well-being can be gained from town planning that promotes more local activity, community inter-reaction and environmentally sound design, thereby leading to a reduction in stress, discomfort and ill-health, especially in the more vulnerable groups. Specifically, the emergent needs from the above brief survey include: the laying out of houses and flats in small groups round local facilities, with all land used as gardens or directly controlled by local groups; the adjustment of building design standards to include greater insulation and better siting; and wider permitted ranges of building size and type, tenure and use. There should be total priority for walking and cycling and local public transport, and local plans should aim for much improved foot- and cycle-ways (as for example in Peterborough and Stevenage). Large units of development which encourage long-distance travel should be restricted or even eliminated.

REFERENCES

Department of Transport, *Transport Statistics, Great Britain: 1978-1988* (London, 1988).

M. Hillman and A. Bollard, *Less Fuel, More Jobs*, Policy Studies Institute, No. 644 (London, 1986).

FURTHER READING

P. Ambrose, *Whatever Happened to Planning?* (London, 1986). A critical review of town planning's failure to meet many needs and of the financial pressures controlling development; proposes some possible (albeit radical) solutions.

M. Bruton (ed.), *The Spirit and Purpose of Planning* (London, 1984). A brief but thorough review of the history and practice of town planning, it particularly examines the role of town planning in current society.

D. Boyle and J. Walker, 'Little Boxes', *Town & Country Planning*, December 1987.

Healthy transport policy

Mayer Hillman

Transport decisions affect the health of the community, but this is poorly recognised. Current policy in the UK focuses mainly on catering for motorised transport, the use of which is often directly or indirectly detrimental to well-being. Its influence can be seen in several ways: physically, owing to death and injury in road accidents; psychologically, in distress due to accidents and the fear of accidents; pathologically, as the pollution and noise from motor vehicles are a source of disease and mental impairment; ecologically, as the exhaust emissions from traffic are a major contributor to global warming, which is highly deleterious to the planet's 'health'.

In terms of the promotion of individual health, the adverse impact of traffic and associated changes in land-use planning deter people from using their feet as a means of travel and thereby discourage them from maintaining physical fitness in this efficient and effective way. Finally, in terms of personal autonomy and self-sufficiency, priority for motorised transport diminishes the ability of people without a car of their own to lead independent lives.

Traffic danger

Road accidents are among the most widely recognised causes of unnecessary suffering from physical injury. Their reduction is an important area of policy on prevention. Each year, over 5,000 people are killed on the roads in incidents involving cars, lorries and motorcycles (Department of Transport, 1989a). A further 90,000, including people involved in accidents not reported to the police but who are treated in hospital, are severely injured.

Comparison of the number of people treated as hospital in-patients after these accidents and the total of all hospital in-patients suggests that the number of beds they occupy is equivalent to the ward capacity of several medium-sized hospitals. In addition, casualty departments have to treat about a third of a million people slightly injured in road accidents each year.

The links observed between social class and mortality and much morbidity (Department of Health and Social Security; Whitehead) are also apparent in road accidents. Such accidents are a primary cause of premature death among children and teenagers, especially those from poor households and neighbourhoods. Whether due to living in a more dangerous environment, that is one with more traffic, to being more dependent on walking, or less likely to be accompanied by an adult, pedestrian fatalities in collisions with motor vehicles are several times higher among children of semi-skilled or unskilled parents than those of professional parents (Office of Population Censuses and Surveys).

Pedestrians and cyclists represent one third of all fatal and serious injuries on the road though they account for only about 7 per cent of all mileage travelled; schoolchildren represent only one in seven of the population but account for a third of all pedestrian and cycle fatalities and serious injuries, mostly as a result of collision with cars; and the riders and passengers of two-wheeled motorised vehicles account for only 1 per cent of personal travel mileage but 20 per cent of all fatal and serious injuries (Department of Transport, 1988, and 1989a).

Calculations made from official statistics reveal that, during any one lifetime, there is a 1 in 2 risk of slight injury, a 1 in 8 risk of serious injury, and a 1 in 150 risk of dying in a road accident. As a result, an average life is shortened by three months due to road fatalities, and a quarter of a million people alive today are likely to die in a road accident (Department of Transport, 1986). Accidents causing death and serious injury have been falling in recent years, but the relative risk by different forms of travel has not stayed constant: for example, the accident rate per mile on a bicycle was five times higher than that by car a decade ago, but it is now over six times higher (Department of Transport, 1989a).

Distress and anxiety

The full extent of the harm caused by road accidents, however, is not limited to those killed or injured. Other people are affected psychologically: when one considers the relatives and friends of those involved in accidents, it is obvious that there are many more victims. Indeed, there are few people who have not had a friend or relative injured in a road accident. Guilt about causing an accident and personal injury is also stressful, particularly if the accident leads to death or disfigurement or if a child is involved. Witnesses also suffer from their experiences.

The death of a close family member is a 'life event' which contributes significantly to survivors' deterioration in health. Studies have shown that the cause of death strongly influences the time it takes for people to become reconciled to their loss, and that the bereaved find it particularly difficult to come to terms with an avoidable death (Parkes). Nor is the harm done necessarily short-term: for many people, recall of the event and grief associated with it, can be a source of distress throughout their life, contributing to a wide range of medical and psychosomatic disorders (Selye). In addition, the loss of the substantial number of domestic pets and wild animals killed and injured in road accidents upsets many people considerably.

There are no statistics to indicate whether there has been any change in the public's anxiety and fear about road accidents. However, the current traffic environment in which a child's perfectly normal momentary lapses of attention can have such a horrific outcome as an 'accidental' death or serious injury does appear to have increasingly encouraged parents to feel that it is unwise to allow their children to travel unaccompanied. Indeed, fear of an accident rather than fear of molestation is the main reason cited by parents for accompanying their children to and from school, and it is a major source of anxiety once children are allowed to travel on their own (Hillman, Henderson and Whalley).

Loss of autonomy

Parents' worry about the dangers of their children being involved in a road accident has led to a situation in which young children can rarely be allowed to get about on their own or to play in the street. Nowadays, most young children are denied that degree of autonomy during an important stage in their development to adulthood because they have to be confined to the home or taken to their destinations in a manner which seldom provides them with the equivalent freedom and exposure to unpredictable experiences enjoyed by their parents and, even more, by their grandparents.

In the early 1970s, on average, children were not allowed by their parents to cross main roads unaccompanied until they had reached the age of eight (although by the age of three or four they can walk reasonable distances), to travel by bus until they were nine, and to cycle on main roads until they were at least ten. Even then, most were discouraged and some not permitted to cycle at all (Hillman, Henderson and Whalley). With the continuing growth of traffic, these restrictions are now much greater.

The consequent loss of a basic freedom for children is reflected in the Department of Transport's National Travel Surveys conducted over the last twenty years, which have shown a marked rise in the incidence of journeys made to escort them. It reflects parents' changing perception of the traffic environment which is increasingly translated in practice into the mother's role in child-rearing being extended to encompass that of accompanier on foot or part-time chauffeur for all the trips children have to make and many of those the children want to make.

Able-bodied mothers accompanying their able-bodied children because of fear is one of the more disturbing and wasteful by-products of the motorised society. It is particularly wasteful as most of these journeys are very time-consuming as they are duplicated, since children have to be taken and collected. A mother, typically with two children, is forced into this tied and potentially unnecessary pattern of activity until the younger child can be granted the parental 'licence' to travel on his or her own.

Other evidence from the most recently published National Travel Survey gives some indication of the extent to which women's lives are affected. In the previous section on town planning, we saw that about one in three households have no car (Department of Transport, 1988). Among people of working age, men are twice as likely as women to be the 'main' driver in a car-owning household and women three times as likely as men not to hold a driving licence.

As a result, women are far more dependent on public transport and walking. Compared with men, they make 50 per cent more journeys by bus, and 40 per cent more on foot. Over the years, both these travel methods have been getting more unpleasant and inconvenient: for the bus user, reliability and hours of operation have declined, and fares have risen much faster than the rate of inflation (Department of Transport, 1989b). For pedestrians, the quality of the local environment has deteriorated as traffic volumes and speed have risen. In addition, surveys have shown that women are increasingly deterred from going out because of fear of being molested. The Home Office *British Crime Survey* recorded that three in five female pensioners, and two in five younger women feel very unsafe walking alone in the dark (Hough and Mayhew).

When compared with *their* parents, many old people too can be seen to have sustained a decline in their capacity to meet their daily travel needs conveniently and safely. Obviously, their well-being is influenced by their ability to maintain social contacts and take part in leisure activities. However, only a minority have use of a car, whilst for the rest, there are now greater demands made on their declining faculties to cope with the speed, ubiquity and severance effects of high volumes of traffic. Old people frequently cite difficulty in crossing roads and fear of traffic as factors influencing their choice of destination and how they travel, even to the extent of limiting their activity outside the home (Hillman, Henderson and Whalley). To compound their problems, their independence has also been reduced by the fact that many of the places they need to reach in their daily lives, such as shops, surgeries and clubs, are no longer within reasonable walking distance. Thus, in common with other people without a car of their own, they are cast in the role of dependants and have to rely on being given a lift to and from their destination or use the same less than adequate public transport system, albeit at free or concessionary rates.

Pollution

Traffic is a major source of noise, widely regarded as disturbing (Hoinville and Prescott-Clarke). This noise can reduce concentration and exacerbate psychiatric disorders. For many people, especially poorer ones living on main roads or for anyone living on flight paths close to airports, it can lead to interrupted sleep (Tarnopolsky, Watkins and Hand). There are adverse effects either if the traffic is continuous, as it then interrupts REM sleep and is subjectively disturbing or, if it is intermittent, as it induces lighter and therefore less restorative sleep (Eberhardt and Akselsson). Surprisingly, there are no surveys of traffic noise levels, but the dramatic rise in the number of motor vehicles on the roads and their spread by area and hour of day and night in the last few decades strongly suggests that these levels, and therefore the harm caused, have increased.

Exhaust fumes from motor vehicles, too, have adverse effects. They contain harmful pollutants which impair efficiency, cause lethargy and headaches, and aggravate some existing medical conditions. They can represent a health risk to pregnant women, young children and old people, all groups in the population which are more sensitive to lower oxygen levels (Lave and Seskin). It is worth noting too that those who are worst-off in society are also more likely to live on main roads and therefore be subject to higher levels of noise and pollution.

The incidence of cancer has been known for many years to be associated with leaded petrol (Blumer and Reich), particularly combined with other carcinogenic substances in vehicle exhaust fumes. Despite recent legislation to reduce the lead content of petrol, it will take several years before safe levels are reached (Jensen and Laxen). Moreover, whilst the amounts of lead and sulphur dioxide from vehicle exhausts are being reduced, those of carbon monoxide, hydrocarbons and nitrogen oxide continue to rise (Department of Transport, 1989b). The benefits of the change in the law requiring new cars to be fitted with catalytic converters from 1992 to reduce these harmful gases will only become markedly apparent later in the decade.

In discussing the environmental hazards associated with growth in the volume of motorised traffic, it is important to highlight what is likely to be the central issue facing policy makers in the very near future. The consensus of expert scientific opinion is that the burning of fossil fuels is likely to lead, within a generation or two, to a destabilising of weather and climate patterns which have evolved over tens of thousands of years unless dramatic reductions are made in the use of such fuels. Transport is a major contributor to greenhouse gases from fuel combustion and, moreover, its share in causing ecological damage in this way is rising.

Lack of exercise

Considerable evidence links low levels of physical exertion with respiratory and heart diseases (Morris, Everitt and Semmence). For most people, walking, if undertaken briskly, and cycling are ideal methods of exercise (Rippe). They encourage the natural use of limbs and lungs and can be associated with varying degrees of effort; they can form part of the daily routine, in contrast to other means of maintaining physical fitness, and are therefore less likely to be abandoned (British Cycling Bureau).

However, existing patterns of travel and land-use militate against people using their legs to get about – on foot or bicycle. A society organised around the use of cars not only discourages car owners from taking these forms of exercise, but indirectly discourages others because of the perceived risk of a road accident, and the lowered quality of the environment for walking and cycling. The adverse consequences of this can be seen in the decisions noted earlier and they are also apparent when older people fail to maintain their fitness because their travel becomes organised around motorised transport.

There are no published statistics on standards of physical fitness, but analysis of data from the National Travel Surveys shows that walking and cycling are declining as travel methods (Hillman). Although cycle ownership is almost as high as car ownership, cycling currently accounts for only

4 per cent of all journeys (Department of Transport, 1988). This remarkably low percentage is no doubt partly explained by the low expenditure by central and local government on cycle networks – the annual equivalent of a few hundred yards of urban motorway.

Transport policy with a health dimension

It is apparent that current transport policy in the UK is deficient in terms of a recognition both of its impact on health and its social context. A transport policy incorporating consideration of the promotion of well-being would not have such undesirable outcomes. These clearly stem from the growing use of means of transport most prejudicial to public health. This use has been encouraged by the transport policies of the last few decades, which have been formulated on the premise that the rising ownership of motorised vehicles, and especially cars, and increases in the capacity of the road network to cater for their use, are indicators of progress. Public expenditure in support of the motor industry and road construction therefore has been high, as has the preference for road rather than rail investment to carry goods. The leniency of existing laws affecting car use and the failure to enforce even these – on such offences as drinking and driving and on speeding – and indulgent tax laws and regulations on company cars and car mileage allowances have clearly contributed to the process.

In the last ten years alone, car mileage has increased by well over 40 per cent. Ironically, people who walk or cycle – the modes most favourable to health – have to do so in an environment which in the main has been rendered progressively unpleasant and unsafe. Moreover, far more motor traffic growth is forecast, and this can only make matters worse. The latest government forecasts predict an increase of between 52 and 86 per cent in volume over the next twenty-five years (Department of Transport, 1989b).

Two sets of practical measures can be taken to give policy a positive health dimension. The first entails reducing the need for motorised travel – with all its attendant adverse impacts – rather than, as at present, generating more demand for it. This could be encouraged, as discussed in the previous section, by planning, land-use and location policies specifically directed towards minimising the distances that have to be travelled to reach shops, schools, sports facilities and so on, and to bring more of the quality of the natural environment into urban areas so that people do not feel so much need to get out to the country for fresh air and tranquility. In addition, policies affecting personal decisions on how and how far to travel need to be framed in such a way as to ensure that proper regard is paid to the wider social and environmental costs of those decisions: at present, these are almost wholly disregarded.

The aim would be to encourage use of those transport modes for personal travel and for the carriage of goods which have the lesser undesirable attributes (Hillman). These policies would enable an increasing proportion of journeys to be made on foot or by bicycle. Safe and convenient networks need to be established for pedestrians, uninterrupted at every road intersection, and for cyclists, either exclusive to them, or shared with motor vehicles subject to low speed limits. Excellent examples of residential environments in which priority is given to pedestrians can be found in Sweden, where the pedestrian casualty rate has been dramatically lowered as a consequence. In the Netherlands, cycle networks have been so successful that well over a quarter of all journeys are made by bicycle and the cycle accident rate is far lower than it is in this country.

In addition, policies on the promotion of public transport, such as those adopted by the South Yorkshire County Council during the 1970s and the Greater London Council in the early 1980s, have shown that low fares can reverse the spiral of increasingly car-dependent activity, and lead to a significant reduction in road accidents (Allsop). Many lessons can be learned from abroad on how to improve the urban environment by promoting new types of shared transport such as light rail and by encouraging the use of rail for freight: in France and Germany nearly three times the proportion of freight is carried on trains compared to Britain, with obvious health and safety benefits.

The second set of measures is concerned with minimising the adverse impacts of motorised travel, in all instances requiring a much higher degree of political commitment to the health-related and social aspects of transport policy than is apparent at present. To reduce accidents and to reduce the fear of accidents – the two objectives are complementary, not synonymous – vehicle speeds can be lowered substantially by using improved enforcement techniques and by imposing more severe penalties for infringements of the traffic law, such as dangerous driving (Plowden and Hillman). Stricter legislation on noise and air pollution can be enacted; random breath testing and lower limits for alcohol in the blood of motorists are further obvious changes that would be beneficial.

Unfortunately, there are insufficient data to calculate the savings to health and welfare services if these sets of measures were adopted. At the least, there exists the prospect of dramatically lowering the number of people who are seriously injured in road accidents each year, and therefore the burden to the NHS of treating them. The reduction in the medical and social pathologies is very likely to lead to further substantial savings as well as to healthier and longer lives for the population.

In recent years, the case for introducing similar sets of measures has been widely urged on governments led by both main political parties. But given the power and influence of organisations with a vested interest in growth in the ownership and use of motor vehicles, this has not happened on a scale that rational policies would suggest. Now, however, major changes in this direction seem highly likely as the imperative need to combat global warming increasingly infiltrates political consciousness. An international programme will have to be agreed during the early 1990s requiring governments to introduce a progressively high 'carbon' tax, which in turn will lead to wider adoption of less space-extensive and motor-dependent patterns of activity. The evidence cited in this chapter strongly indicates that the outcome of such a programme, implemented through transport and planning policies, will very positively enhance public health.

REFERENCES

Richard Allsop, *Fares and road casualties* (London, Greater London Council, 1983).

W. Blumer and T. Reich, 'Leaded gasoline – a cause of cancer', *Environment International,* 3 (1980).

British Cycling Bureau, *Cycling: the healthy alternative* (London, British Cycling Bureau, 1978).

Department of Health and Social Security, *Inequalities in Health*. The Black Report (London, DHSS, 1980).

Department of Transport, *Road Accidents in Great Britain 1985: The Casualty Report* (London, 1986).

Department of Transport, *National Travel Survey 1985/86 Report* (London, 1988).

Department of Transport, *Road Accidents Great Britain, 1988: The Casualty Report* (London, 1989a).

Department of Transport, *Transport Statistics Great Britain, 1978-1988* (London, 1989b).

J. Eberhardt and K. R. Akselsson, 'The Influences of Continuous and Intermittent Traffic Noise on Sleep', *Journal of Sound and Vibration*, 114 (1987).

Mayer Hillman, Irwin Henderson and Anne Whalley, *Transport Realities and Planning Policy* (London, Political and Economic Planning (now Policy Studies Institute), 1976).

Mayer Hillman, 'Walking and Cycling: Planning for the Green Modes. A Critique of Public Policy and Practice', in R.S. Tolley (ed.), *The Greening of Urban Transport: Planning for Walking and Cycling in Western Cities* (London, 1990).

Gerald Hoinville and Patricia Prescott-Clarke, *Traffic Disturbance and Amenity Values* (London, Social Community and Planning Research, 1978).

Mike Hough and Pat Mayhew, *Taking Account of Crime: Key Findings from the Second British Crime Survey*, Home Office Research Study No. 85 (London, 1985).

R.A. Jensen and D.P.H. Laxen, 'The Effect of the Phase-down of Lead in Petrol on Levels of Lead in Air', *The Science of the Total Environment*, 59 (1987).

Lester Lave and Eugene Seskin, *Air Pollution and Human Health* (Baltimore, 1977).

J.N. Morris, M.G. Everitt and A.M. Semmence, 'Coronary Heart Disease and Exercise', *Health Trends*, 19 (1987).

Office of Population Censuses and Surveys, *Occupational Mortality, 1970-72*, Series DS No. 1 (London, 1978).

Colin Murray Parkes, *Bereavement: Studies of Grief in Adult Life* (London, 1972).

Stephen Plowden and Mayer Hillman, *Danger on the Road: the Needless Scourge* (London, Policy Studies Institute, 1984).

James M. Rippe et al, 'Walking for Health and Fitness', *Journal of the American Medical Association*, 259, 18 (1988).

Hans Selye, *Stress of Life* (London, 1957).

Alex Tarnopolsky, Gareth Watkins and David Hand, 'Aircraft Noise and Mental Health: Prevalence of Individual Symptoms', *Psychological Medicine*, 10 (1980).

M. Whitehead, *The Health Divide: Inequalities in Health in the 1980s* (London, Health Education Council, 1987).

FURTHER READING

Stephen Plowden and Mayer Hillman, *Danger on the Road: the Needless Scourge* (London, Policy Studies Institute, 1984).

British Cycling Bureau, *Cycling: the healthy alternative* (London, 1978). Ten papers on medical, social and planning aspects of cycling and health.

National Consumer Council, *What's Wrong with Walking?* (London, 1987).

Mayer Hillman, John Adams and John Whitelegg, *One False Move . . . A Study of Children's Independent Mobility* (London, Policy Studies Institute, 1991).

Mayer Hillman, *The Resource Conscious Society* (London, Policy Studies Institute, 1991).

Tim Elkin and Duncan McLaren with Mayer Hillman, *Reviving the City* (London, Friends of the Earth with Policy Studies Institute, 1991).

CHAPTER 5

Enemies of the people

Our consideration of some adverse environments for health concludes with studies of three of the malign influences exerted by some trading organisations and banks: the tobacco pushers, the arms traders, and the moneylenders who encouraged a mountain of Third World debts to the rich countries.

The tobacco pushers
Patti White

One consumer product is so exceptionally dangerous that an estimated quarter of its regular users are killed by it. The product is, of course, cigarettes. These little tubes of chopped up vegetation kill about 2.5 million people annually (Chandler). In Britain about 100,000 people will die annually, into the 1990s at least, because they were smokers. An equivalent number of lives would be lost if the entire population of a city the size of Oxford were wiped out every year.

The magnitude of the tobacco epidemic is difficult to comprehend. Perhaps this is partly because it is so common a cause of death. Certainly the news media focus on life's more dramatic events, effectively diverting the public's attention from the quieter tobacco epidemic. At a time of widespread fear about AIDS and the use of illicit drugs, this is perhaps understandable. Yet even in the United States, where mortality from AIDS is much higher and death rates from tobacco-induced diseases like lung cancer are lower than in Britain, tobacco smoking causes more premature deaths than do AIDS, cocaine, heroin, alcohol, fire, automobile accidents, homicide and suicide all put together (Warner). This is not to say that tobacco necessarily presents a more critical health problem than these other causes of early death – each has its own social and personal consequences which make a nonsense of comparisons – but it does put the scale of the tobacco epidemic into some perspective.

The scientific community has been aware for more than thirty years that tobacco is highly dangerous. Serious attempts to inform the public about the danger date back to at least 1962, when the first of four Royal College of Physicians' reports on smoking was published. Since then, smoking has declined dramatically. In the late 1950s over half of British adults smoked cigarettes, while about one in three does so today. Yet there are still 13 million adults who smoke cigarettes. So what keeps them smoking?

There are three broad reasons why we as a nation spent about £7 billion on tobacco in 1988. Although demand has fallen dramatically in Britain, smokers continue to need tobacco; there is a powerful industry that continues to promote and sell tobacco; and governments have become too habituated to the revenue from tobacco to frame effective policies to discourage its use.

A habit that dies hard

Although more than two-thirds of smokers say that they want to stop and even more have tried at least once to do so, the habit is hard to break. The director of the US National Institute on Drug Abuse made headlines in 1985 when he characterised nicotine as society's 'most prevalent drug of abuse', and more resistant to treatment than heroin. For both the manufacturer and the Treasury that is good news: it means that even if times get tough the smoker is more likely to go without cornflakes or floor polish than fags and Chancellors of the Exchequer can put up the tax without losing revenue.

'Dealing in addictive drugs is not a crime of passion or hot blood but a cold-blooded, premeditated act by people who know the drugs can kill', Kenneth Clarke MP told the Conservative Party Conference in 1984. The then junior Health Minister was speaking about heroin. Tobacco is a greater generator of wealth and ill-health; it also generates for its manufacturers an inconvenient but obviously not insuperable drawback. Six companies dominate the transnational tobacco industry and they are among the richest and most powerful transnationals in the world. Although they are diversifying rapidly into food, drink, financial services, retailing and other wide-ranging interests, making cigarettes remains their most profitable activity. Over a decade ago annual worldwide sales stood somewhere around four trillion and were worth more than $40 billion (United Nations Conference on Trade and Development). More recent estimates are that the world's one billion smokers consume five trillion cigarettes a year (Chandler). Nor is the end of the road for the tobacco companies anywhere in sight. While smoking rates are decreasing in some industrialised countries, in the developing world tobacco consumption is increasing rapidly.

These populous countries, many already burdened with problems of mal-nutrition and communicable diseases, offer rich pickings.

The 'controversy' smokescreen

To get a true picture of the industry's ethical position, one must remind oneself that it has never publicly acknowledged that smoking is even dangerous. It refers to the more than 50,000 scientific investigations that have demonstrated beyond question the hazards of tobacco as 'the smoking and health controversy'. Commenting on the fifteenth annual report on smoking published by the US Surgeon General in 1979, Philip Morris, the makers of Marlboro, said, despite the money and effort poured into research, that 'no conclusive medical or clinical proof has been discovered . . . the tobacco industry continues to maintain the controversy can be resolved only by medical and scientific knowledge' (Wilkinson). It would be difficult to imagine what the manufacturers would consider 'conclusive' evidence of the harm done. But their statement should not be taken at face value: it was, of course, a smokescreen used to imply that the industry is just as interested as everyone else at getting to the 'truth'. Their position, which with time looks increasingly inane, is intended to assuage smokers' doubts about the risks they are taking.

The industry defends its flouting of the evidence by saying that it is 'merely statistical', yet the industry's paid apologists rely on 'mere statistical evidence' to try to prove that advertising has no effect on tobacco consumption. They are quick, too, to try to take advantage of any statistics that might enhance their case. Alas, they are not always scrupulous in this practice.

An example of the industry's tactics occurred on 20 June 1986, when *The Times* newspaper misreported the results of a forthcoming paper in the *British Journal of Cancer*. Under the headline, 'Passive smoking: no significant danger', the newspaper said that new research conducted at the Institute of Cancer Research had 'the hallmark of turning the received wisdom' on the hazards of breathing other people's tobacco smoke 'into one of the medical controversies of the year'. The industry was not slow to capitalise on the mistake of *The Times*: the Tobacco Advisory Council, the industry's trade organisation, circulated a copy of the article to all MPs saying that it would 'add a valuable dimension to this public issue and put it into perspective'. Within days the transnational tobacco companies had shared the prize and the same *Times* article was being used in industry advertising in Australia to question the need to restrict smoking in public places.

In an attempt to rectify *The Times*' mistake, Professor Robin Weiss, director of the Institute of Cancer Research, and Professor Julian Peto, its chief epidemiologist, wrote to the newspaper pointing out that the Institute had only collaborated on the research, which had been funded by the Tobacco Advisory Council, and that the results, far from contradicting previous findings, tended to confirm them. Professor Weiss reportedly asked the Tobacco Advisory Council to retract the extremely misleading information it had circulated to MPs and local authorities, but his request went unanswered (Anon. a).

Wealth not health

On the face of it, governments entrusted with the public well-being should be formulating policies to make it easier for people to decide not to smoke. In fact, most governments come to rely upon the apparent economic benefit from tobacco. These include the large amounts of money smokers pay in tobacco taxes, handouts from the industry to sports and the arts and the savings on pensions for smokers who die prematurely. Countries in which the industry provides employment through tobacco farming or manufacture have an additional disincentive to control tobacco use. In Britain, successive governments' responses to the tobacco epidemic have been inadequate. Cabinet papers now being released under the thirty-year rule reveal just how government has failed to keep the well-being of the public as its primary goal.

As early as 1956, the Health Minister, Robert Turton, was urged by the Standing Medical Advisory Committee to 'inform the public of the known connection between smoking and cancer of the lung and the risks involved in heavy smoking'. At the time, the Medical Research Council's chairman described the statistical association found between smoking and the incidence of lung cancer as 'so massive as to be incontrovertible' (Anon. b).

When a special Cabinet sub-committee set up under R.A. 'Rab' Butler to produce a government statement on tobacco reported to Cabinet on 1 May 1956, Butler recommended that 'any statement on this subject should not involve the government too deeply in responsibility for dealing with the possible consequences of excessive smoking'. The statement finally prepared for the Health Minister noted the spectacular rise in lung cancer incidence that had occurred over the previous twenty-five years, but put the findings 'in perspective' by emphasising that more men died from strokes and apoplexies (Anon. c).

It is misleading to speak of government policy on tobacco, as no comprehensive policy exists. The reality is that each government department acts to satisfy its own internal demands and these objectives often fail to coincide with those of the Department of Health.

The department with perhaps the greatest interest in tobacco is the Treasury, which collected £6 billion in tobacco taxes for the year 1988-89 (Hansard, 1990). Tobacco is the Chancellor's third largest source of consumer revenue after VAT and hydrocarbon oil (Taylor). It can be clearly demonstrated that sharp tax increases make tobacco consumption go down. But because many smokers will continue to smoke despite higher prices, the higher revenue brought in by tax increases offsets the fall in consumption. Indeed, the effect of price on consumption has encouraged health advocates to campaign for steady tobacco tax increases. Sharp increases, however, have a drawback for the government: inflation. Tobacco is a component of the Retail Price Index and any significant increase in its price will be reflected there.

The industry has never been a massive employer in Britain because tobacco manufacture is highly mechanised. In these days of increasing automation the number of employees is declining – from about 35,000 when the Conservatives came to power in 1979 to about 13,000 today (Hansard, 1987a, b, 1988). The Departments of Employment and Trade and Industry are involved in tobacco through their interest in maintaining existing jobs and creating new ones, especially in areas of high unemployment. In Northern Ireland alone, the government has paid over £33 million toward the maintenance and development of the industry since 1980 (Hansard, 1989). One hardly needs to point out the incompatibility of this policy with the policies of the Health Department or to contrast the size of this sum with the meagre handouts to ASH (Action on Smoking and Health), the Health Education Authority and SHEG (Scottish Health Education Group) for funding anti-tobacco information programmes.

Other government departments have a less obvious but no less compelling interest in tobacco. The ministries responsible for sports and the arts, the Ministry of Sport in the Department of the Environment and the Office of Arts and Libraries, want to increase business sponsorship in their respective domains. Tobacco companies, needing desperately to boost their public image, are anxious to comply. They need to provide sponsorship, since this gives access to television promotion. Advertisements for cigarettes, but not those for other tobacco products, have been banned from television since 1965, using powers taken under the Independent Broadcasting Act, 1964. Sports sponsorship in particular is an excellent method of getting the tobacco pushers' message across to a wide audience, especially to the most important target of tomorrow's smokers – children.

Governments have another powerful reason to take no action to curb tobacco use. The simple fact is that if fewer people smoke, more will survive long enough to collect their pensions. Looked at cynically, tobacco very conveniently kills off a lot of people in their late middle age, a time when they are reaching the end of their economically productive life anyway. This was clearly brought out in a 1971 government inquiry that included officials from the Treasury, Customs and Excise, the Department of Trade and Industry and the Department of Health and Social Security. Their report was never published, but a copy was passed to *The Guardian* newspaper which printed details of it in 1980.

The inquiry estimated that a reduction in smoking of 20 per cent over a thirty-year period would result in a saving of a quarter of a million lives by the turn of the century. Although there would be savings on health costs in the short term, this would be offset by £12 million in increased social security payments by the year 2000. Years ago the American civil rights movement used a catchphrase that characterises Britain's situation today with regard to the lethal habit of smoking. It ran: 'If you're not part of the solution, you're part of the problem'. Many parts of the community, in serving their own interests, collaborate with the tobacco industry to keep Britons smoking and dying.

Tobacco's allies and accomplices

The industry's most powerful allies in Britain are the one hundred or so MPs estimated to support it actively (Taylor). They include some paid parliamentary consultants who do much of the political lobbying. There are others who have vested interests, including MPs who have a legitimate constituency interest, such as a tobacco factory's employees among their constituents. MPs may also have private interests in advertising or public relations agencies that represent tobacco companies, or in firms such as newspapers and magazines that benefit from tobacco advertising.

Other institutions and individuals collude with the industry in a less direct but nonetheless influential way. By accepting sponsorship money some of society's most valued institutions, such as sports associations, television organisations, theatres, opera and ballet companies and or-chestras, tacitly show their approval of tobacco. The tobacco industry's image has become slightly tarnished, however, by criticism of television companies for their inability to control blatant tobacco television adver-tising through sports sponsorship. In 1986, more than 360 hours of tobacco-sponsored sport was shown on television, 99 per cent of it by the BBC (Roberts). Reacting to widespread criticism of this practice, the IBA announced that it would no longer carry tobacco-sponsored events and the BBC tightened its procedure for broadcasting such events.

Shifts in acceptability

There are other indications that the industry's silent collaborators are defecting. More and more local governments are rejecting tobacco advertising on council-owned sites. After the thirty deaths in the 1987 fire at Kings Cross station, London Regional Transport banned tobacco ads from the Underground and extended its no smoking rule. Other transport authorities also restricted smoking and in a growing number of workplaces, cinemas and other public places the same trend is evident.

This trend for institutions to adapt themselves to the needs of the non-smoking majority is the most striking feature of a shift in the social acceptability of smoking in Britain. The advance has been gained by the action of anti-tobacco advocacy groups, by research revealing the harm done by passive smoking and by consumer demand for more smoke-free space.

Public interest groups such as ASH have persistently drawn attention to the ineffectiveness of the agreements the tobacco industry has made with governments on advertising and promotion. They have also laboured to establish that not smoking is normal social behaviour and that the non-smoker's right to breathe clean air must supersede that of the smoker to create environmental pollution.

Such attempts to encourage the public to view tobacco in a more realistic light received an enormous fillip in 1984 when the BMA put the weight of its prestige and its sophisticated public relations skills behind the anti-tobacco campaign. The pressure created by the BMA's example has propelled other groups toward an advocacy role.

Although these groups are encouraging changes in the general perception of smoking, more important has been the public demand for cleaner air. It is now considered reasonable for non-smokers to expect to be free from the discomfort of other people's tobacco smoke and, naturally enough, as the number of non-smokers grows, the justice of their expectations seems irrefutable. Increases in smoke-free areas promote decreases in tobacco consumption simply because smokers have fewer opportunities to light up. Many are encouraged to quit altogether. And as the habit becomes less acceptable, its veneer of sophistication is gradually stripped away, as is the illusion that it is a normal part of adult life.

The image of tobacco and the transnational companies that produce it is becoming even worse as people grow more environmentally aware. Tobacco smoke is, unsurprisingly, the main source of indoor air pollution; it has been estimated that the risk of lung cancer from passive smoking is some fifty to a hundred times greater than the risk of lung cancer from exposure to asbestos particles in buildings that contain asbestos materials (Doll and Peto). Smoking also produces a lot of rubbish. The Tidy Britain

Campaign estimates that one-third of the litter on Britain's streets is from smoking materials. Much more serious, however, are global concerns about tobacco growing and curing.

Tobacco curing requires an extraordinary amount of energy. While gas or oil is used in industrialised countries, these sources of energy are too expensive for many developing countries, where wood is used instead. For every 300 cigarettes made a tree is burnt. That means that for each acre of tobacco flue-cured by wood, an acre of woodland disappears (Muller). This has already led to a timber shortage in some parts of Africa and the potentially disastrous environmental consequences are all too clear.

Awareness of the global costs of tobacco has led development and environmental groups, such as Friends of the Earth, to add their voice to those who advocate better policies on tobacco control. This is the most promising development for ending the tobacco epidemic. It is only by forming a broad-based coalition of public interest groups that the necessity for rational public policy and government action can be articulated and a solution pursued. Governments are under too many conflicting pressures, and health departments generally command too low a priority, to ensure that appropriate and effective policies will be framed and implemented without widespread public support. Equally, a loud and articulate voice is needed to speak out against the tobacco pushers and against policies that do nothing to discourage its use. In a world where advertising and sponsorship of sports and cultural events constantly reinforce the social acceptability of smoking, and where the wealth of the tobacco industry gives it a degree of access to decision makers that can only be envied by pro-health forces, the only counterpoint likely to lead society out of the epidemic is the voice and example of such a coalition.

REFERENCES

Anon. a, 'Fag ends', *Private Eye*, 15 May 1987.
Anon. b, 'Cancer and Smoking Issue Fudged', *The Independent*, 2 January 1987.
Anon. c, 'Ministers Threw Smokescreen over Tobacco Risks', *New Scientist*, 8 January 1987.
W. Chandler, *Worldwatch Paper 68: Banishing Tobacco* (Washington, Worldwatch Institute, 1986).
R. Doll and J. Peto, 'Passive Smoking', *British Journal of Cancer*, 54 (1986).
House of Commons Hansard, 1989/90 Session. Col. 713 (8/2/90).
House of Commons Hansard, 1988/89 Session. Vol. 140, Col. 421 (14/11/88).
House of Commons Hansard, 1988/89 Session. Vol. 149, Col. 138 (14/3/89).
House of Commons Hansard, a, 1986/87 Session. Vol. 123, No. 58, Col. 692 (3/12/87).
House of Commons Hansard, b, 1986/87 Session. Vol. 108, No. 36, Col. 567-68 (22/1/87).
M. Muller, *Tomorrow's Epidemic* (London, War on Want, 1978).
J. Roberts, *The Name of the Game* (Manchester, Project Smoke Free, 1986).
P. Taylor, *The Smoke Ring: Tobacco, Money and Multinational Politics* (London, 1985).

United Nations Conference on Trade and Development, *Marketing and Distribution of Tobacco* (Geneva, UN, 1978).

K. Warner, 'Health and Economic Implications of a Tobacco-free Society', *Journal of the American Medical Association*, 258 (1987).

R. Weiss and J. Peto, 'Disputed risk of passive smoking', *The Times*, 5 July 1986.

J. Wilkinson, *Tobacco; The Facts Behind the Smokescreen* (Harmondsworth, 1986).

FURTHER READING

H. Ashton and R. Stepney, *Smoking: Psychology and Pharmacology* (London, 1982). Still the most enlightening and readable account of the psychological and pharmacological determinants of smoking.

B. Jacobson, *Beating the Ladykillers: Women and Smoking* (London 1986). Explores why women are a special target for tobacco promotion.

P. Taylor, *The Smoke Ring: Tobacco, Money and Multinational Politics* (London, 1985). The definitive work on the politics of tobacco – indispensable.

U. Ram Nath, *Smoking: Third World Alert* (Oxford, 1986). The basic facts concerning the tobacco epidemic now being exported to developing countries.

R. Roemer, *Legislative Action to Combat the World Smoking Epidemic* (Geneva, WHO, 1982) and *Recent Developments in Legislation to Combat the World Smoking Epidemic* (Geneva, WHO, 1986). Brave attempts at an unwieldy subject, these two volumes are useful guides to worldwide legislative action on tobacco.

Royal College of Physicians, *Smoking and Health Now, a Report of the Royal College of Physicians* (London, 1983). This and the preceding three Royal College reports on smoking are the lay person's best introduction to the medical case against tobacco.

US Surgeon General, *Smoking and Health*, a Report of the Surgeon General, US Department of Health, Education and Welfare. Annual reports from 1964. These are admirable technical summaries and reviews of the literature on tobacco.

The 'Smoke-Free Europe Series' is a collection of ten booklets from WHO Regional Office for Europe. One describes WHO's programme for building networks in Europe to promote effective public health policies on tobacco; each of the remaining nine addresses a particular aspect of tobacco policy. Intended for the non-specialist reader, the booklets give a concise and current view of a particular tobacco control issue. Available on request from WHO's Regional Office for Europe, 8 Scherfigsvej, DK-2100 Copenhagen, Denmark. Available in English, French, German and Russian. Also available: *It Can be Done: A Smoke-Free Europe* (Geneva, WHO, 1990).

The arms traders

Steve Webster

Concern over the damaging effects of the armaments business is hardly new, yet the world continues to spend vast amounts on arms. The dramatic change in relations between East and West has brought major progress in disarmament negotiations and cuts in the defence expenditures of NATO and Warsaw Pact countries now seem likely. However, these positive developments are set in the context of the world's massive military expenditure, which now exceeds $900,000 million per annum. At the heart of this spending is the purchase of military hardware from the arms industries which supply everything from tanks and missiles to guns and grenades: hardware which at best will never be used and at worst will kill, maim and destroy.

Much has been said about the likely effects of nuclear war and its horrific consequences for health, but the arms business already seriously damages the lives of hundreds of millions of people. As Bernard Lown, co-president of International Physicians for the Prevention of Nuclear War, said:

> One hour's global military expenditure would more than suffice to immunize the 3.5 million children destined to die annually from preventable infectious diseases. James Grant, Director of UNICEF, has posed the question whether the world would tolerate a Hiroshima-like catastrophe every three days. This, in fact, is now happening, for every three days 120,000 children die unnecessarily – the very toll of casualties following the atomic bombing of Hiroshima. Indeed the children of the world are already living in the rubble of World War III. (Sivard, 1986, p. 3).

This case study examines the role of the weapons business in this continuing catastrophe. To demonstrate some of the effects of this business, the study looks first at aspects of the international trade in arms.

The Iran-Iraq war . . . and many others

The Iran-Iraq war provided a graphic and tragic illustration of the end result of the arms business. In stark figures, between 1980 and 1988 the conflict resulted in the deaths of over a million people. Over 100,000 civilians died and many more were seriously injured. In one way or another the war deeply affected the lives of everyone in both countries – few families escaped tragedy.

Sadly the war served to demonstrate the phenomenally destructive power of so-called 'conventional' weapons. Yet in the face of the devastation, many arms companies were only too keen to supply the weapons 'needs' of the warring parties – and with the support and approval of their own governments. By 1987 the Stockholm International Peace Research Institute (SIPRI) had identified some fifty-three countries which had supplied arms to the two combatants; these included all the chief arms exporting countries. At least twenty-six countries are known to have supplied equipment to both sides during the war, including Britain.

Thus the conflict was cynically exploited by the arms traders – keen to make up for a relative decline in sales to Third World countries (many now deeply in debt). Not only did the arms traders profit directly from the misery of others, but their involvement had a major impact on the course of the war itself. Without their continuing supplies of weapons and spare parts the war would almost certainly have ground to a halt much sooner.

Unfortunately the Iran-Iraq war was no isolated example – armaments are often used for the purpose for which they are designed. Between 1945 and 1989 there were 127 wars around the world, resulting in an estimated twenty-two million war-related deaths. The great majority of these conflicts have taken place in Third World countries, well away from the industrialised nations which have been only too willing to supply the arms. In this context, any claims that armaments have helped to keep the peace seem questionable, to say the least.

Figures alone cannot hope to convey the true horror of war. For each person killed, many others are injured, bereaved or made homeless. Many are forced to flee for their lives, becoming refugees with little or no means of supporting either themselves or their families. Economies are ruined and lives shattered. There is often massive damage to the environment – homes, crops and livestock destroyed. The destructive power of modern weaponry is such that vast areas may be laid waste – made uninhabitable for years to come. Food production may suffer severely, with the inevitable death toll through malnutrition when war occurs in the poorer countries. The catalogue of damage goes on and on.

The weapons trade

The international arms trade is big business – valued at over $40,000 million per annum. However, the trade in major items of military equipment such as aircraft, tanks, ships and missiles (often referred to as 'major weapons') is dominated by a handful of countries. These are the United States, the Soviet Union, France, Britain, West Germany, China and Italy; they account for over 90 per cent of all exports of such weaponry.

It is commonly thought that the arms trade is synonymous with shady deals and illegal gun-running. While such activities certainly do take place, the overall picture is rather different. In practice arms transfers are largely controlled and approved by governments, with the weapons supplies being dominated by the major arms manufacturing companies.

While arms deals are generally between a company and the government of a recipient country, exports can usually go ahead only with the approval of the government of the supplying country; this applies particularly to sales of 'major weapons'. All the leading supplying countries have well-defined export controls; certainly most of the military equipment exported from Britain is sold with either the direct or indirect approval of government. It would, however, be a mistake to interpret the existence of such controls as a commitment to reducing arms exports; rather they are used to ensure that arms serve the demands of government policy (particularly foreign and defence policy).

So where does all this hardware go? Over two-thirds of the international arms trade is accounted for by the weapons purchases of developing countries. The picture is dominated by the Middle East, which takes around half of all weapons bought by developing countries. For simplicity the phrase 'developing countries' is here used to describe all countries not regarded as developed; it therefore includes the world's very poorest countries which many regard as underdeveloped rather than developing. In 1983-87 the five leading arms importing countries amongst developing countries were: Iraq, India, Egypt, Syria and Saudi Arabia.

The main arms suppliers are often only too happy to provide weapons to countries involved in regional conflicts, thus encouraging regional arms races. They appear to be much less interested in working for the resolution of such conflicts, and encouraging and enabling the countries involved to reduce their military spending. This is clearly illustrated by the sheer scale of arms sales to the Middle East and the appalling example of military sales to the combatants during the Iran-Iraq war.

Developing countries

For the world's poorer countries military expenditure, including the cost of imported military hardware, has alarming social effects. This is not because they spend vast amounts on the military compared with the much richer industrialised countries (the opposite is the case), but rather that they can ill afford the expenditure that is devoted to the military.

Poverty in the developing world already exacts a tremendous toll; for example, one person in five is undernourished. Yet over the last two decades there has been a dramatic increase in the military expenditure of developing countries, particularly on arms purchases. In 1987, for example, these countries spent over $30,000 million on arms imports. In many countries, money spent on the acquisition of military hardware consumes scarce resources which are desperately needed to provide adequate food supplies, decent housing or basic education and health care services. Weapons purchases have also played a significant role in exacerbating the debt problems of developing countries.

Africa provides a graphic illustration of the social impact of military spending. As in many other parts of the world, the continent's military expenditure far outweighs spending on health services. In 1986, for example, African countries spent three times as much on the military as they did on health services: military expenditure was $12,950 million, compared with health spending of just $4,295 million (Sivard, 1989, p. 49; Egypt is not included in the analysis of African countries).

Africa's urgent need for improved health care rather than more military hardware imported from the rich industrialised countries is highlighted by these few examples of figures for 1986:

* Only 31 per cent of the population has reasonable access to a safe and adequate water supply.
* The infant mortality rate is 108 (108 deaths under one year, for every 1000 live births, i.e. more than one child in ten dies before reaching its first birthday).
* Average life expectancy is just 51 years, whereas in Western Europe it is 73 years.
* There is just one doctor for every 7561 people, in Western Europe there is one for every 495.

All of these figures are averages for the whole of Africa – in many countries the position is far worse (Sivard, 1989, pp. 50-5).

Human rights

Arms sales also play their part in the violation of civil and political human rights when unpopular repressive regimes buy weapons to maintain their positions through armed force. An alarming number of countries are subject to military rule, and over fifty developing countries now have military-controlled governments. Military regimes frequently use 'repressive technology' – guns, 'riot-control' equipment, armoured vehicles, surveillance devices and the like – against their own population in attempts to maintain control and suppress dissent.

Repression means that dissidents are imprisoned, tortured or even murdered. Many prisoners are badly treated and torture often results in long-lasting physical and psychological damage. Relatives and friends of victims suffer too. There is, for example, the appalling plight of the families of the people who have been made to 'disappear' – not knowing if the victim has fallen prey to the death squads or is languishing in some anonymous prison cell.

Repression is strongly linked to poverty and underdevelopment – the priorities of authoritarian governments often bear little relation to the needs of large sections of their populations. Militarised regimes are far more likely to acquire new weapons systems or counter-insurgency gear rather than invest in new health care facilities, the training of sufficient medical staff, or even the provision of adequate food supplies.

Britain and the arms trade

So where does Britain fit into the picture? The UK is one of the world's four leading arms exporters and British weaponry is sold throughout the world – chiefly to developing countries. Its position in the 1980s was boosted by major export deals with Saudi Arabia which included the sale of Tornado strike aircraft – the very latest military technology.

At the centre of this trade are the British government and the arms industry. It is the government that regulates the trade, yet at the same time actively promotes arms exports. However, it is the arms industry that is responsible for manufacturing the weaponry and for continuing to invest resources in the arms trade. One of the most important ways in which the two work together is through the Defence Export Services Organisation (DESO) – a department within the Ministry of Defence. The role of the DESO is to promote overseas sales of British military equipment. For example, it organises major exhibitions such as the British Army Equipment Exhibition and the Royal Navy Equipment Exhibition, each of which attracts several hundred companies keen to export their hardware and potential buyers from dozens of overseas countries.

In common with the other chief arms exporting countries Britain continues to sell weaponry to conflict areas and to repressive regimes. In particular, it has sold military equipment to both Iran and Iraq simultaneously and continued with major sales to many other countries in the region, notably Saudi Arabia. Many of Britain's customers are authoritarian regimes with bad human rights records, such as Indonesia. In the 1980s for example, Britain was an important supplier of weapons to the repressive Pinochet regime in Chile; this was in spite of public pressure on the government to reinstate the ban on arms sales to Chile imposed by the Labour government in the mid 1970s. Britain is thought to be one of the world's leading suppliers of 'repressive technology' – equipment which is used directly in the suppression of political dissent.

The big spenders

It is the developed world that is responsible for the lion's share of global military expenditure – over 80 per cent of the total. Not surprisingly this has been concentrated within NATO and Warsaw Pact countries – the chief arms-producing countries are themselves the chief consumers of military hardware. In Britain, the Ministry of Defence is the arms companies' main customer; more weaponry is sold to the ministry than goes overseas, accounting for over two-thirds of the arms manufactured in Britain.

In Britain, the government has been spending on the military an amount similar to its spending on health services. Over 40 per cent of the Ministry of Defence's annual budget is spent on new military hardware. The projected cost of the new Trident nuclear weapons system now under construction is around £10,000 million – compare that with the cost of providing new community health centres or cutting hospital waiting lists. The military sector also consumes a colossal proportion of all resources devoted to research and development. Around half of all government-funded research and development in Britain is devoted to military projects. Yet many other areas of the economy are screaming out for adequate research funding.

The arms industry has a massive vested interest in the continuance of high levels of military spending and arms exports, regardless of the effects. It acts as a powerful lobby for incessant militarisation and has a major impact on the way in which governments in the developed world perceive the 'need' for yet more weapons purchases. Thus it also acts as a major pressure against the serious pursuit of arms control/disarmament agreements.

The lessening of East/West tensions is, however, weakening the position of many arms manufacturers in the industrialised countries. This is enhanced by their difficulty in arguing that arms production is of wider benefit to the community – the old claim that the arms industry is 'good for jobs' is now in tatters. In Britain the number of people involved in arms production has fallen dramatically over the last twenty years. Even in the export sector, the number of jobs supported both directly and indirectly by arms exports has fallen. Certainly money invested in other areas of the economy would help to create and support more jobs than in the military sector. In the US, for example, it has been estimated that military expenditures generate 50 per cent fewer jobs than if similar amounts were spent on servicing people's needs such as health care or education (US Bureau of Labor Statistics).

The threat of war

Probably the greatest threat which ultimately is posed by the arms business to humanity's health and well-being is the potential cost of conventional or nuclear war in the northern hemisphere. The nuclear arms race has already consumed massive resources, but the worst threat of all comes from the possibility of nuclear war. In the words of the Alternative Defence Commission:

It has become impossible to quantify the enormities of a nuclear exchange. In addition to the lethal effects of the blast, heat and radiation, many millions of people in combatant and non-combatant countries would die from disease and starvation as the world's economy and agricultural production collapse. In addition, recent scientific research indicates that a large nuclear war could have a drastic effect on the world's climate. Cooling and reductions in sunlight could cause massive crop failures and general ecological catastrophe. Such a nuclear winter would threaten the survival of the remainder of the world's population (p. 2).

The threat goes still further. A non-nuclear war would also result in tremendous devastation through the massive destructive power of modern 'conventional' weapons, which was demonstrated in Vietnam and Kampuchea. On top of all this there are the horrendous effects of chemical and biological warfare.

Alternatives

A constantly recurring theme has been the reluctance of those involved in the arms business – directly or indirectly – to explore non-military solutions to conflict. The arms manufacturers' vested interest is obvious – but it is governments that ultimately bear the burden of responsibility. The present progress in disarmament negotiations between the US and the Soviet Union demonstrates that major progress can be made once the political will is there. Problems which have obstructed talks for years are suddenly being overcome.

There are many avenues through which peaceful solutions can be sought over and above bilateral talks between the two superpowers. The United Nations was created to put an end to the scourge of war. Its Security Council is supposed to facilitate peaceful resolution of conflicts, but so often the major arms-producing countries have acted to obstruct peaceful change. The UN arms embargo on South Africa, which could have become a positive demonstration of such an approach, was undermined by the willingness of the chief western arms exporters to continue transfers of military technology and know-how to Pretoria.

More is required than simply pressing countries to enter into meaningful negotiations. There is a need for a different approach to the whole issue of defence – a need to explore alternative defence strategies. In Britain, the Alternative Defence Commission has produced reports exploring viable non-nuclear defence policies. In *Without the Bomb* a central proposal is that Britain should adopt a non-provocative defence policy – one that concentrates strictly on deterring potential attacks rather than threatening a potential opponent. The report said:

> Every defence policy involves risks; none can offer foolproof guarantees of security. However, the risks of 'defensive deterrence' are not as great as those of nuclear deterrence. By its very nature, defensive deterrence would tend to reduce tension and thus the likelihood of war being launched by mistake or of pressures towards pre-emption. And, if deterrence should fail, the war would be less destructive. (p. xvi)

This approach is also highly relevant to non-nuclear disarmament, for a defending country does not need to match an aggressor's military force.

Military thinkers often assume that something like a three-to-one numerical (or some equivalent) advantage is needed by the side taking the offensive in war. As a defensive strategy requires merely that one's forces are strong enough to frustrate an attack, they do not need to be as numerous or as powerful. (Alternative Defence Commission, p. 7)

Finally

It is the developed world that should be made to shoulder the responsibility for the effects of the arms business. The changing climate between East and West is to be welcomed, but pressure for change must continue. This is no time for complacency – the proposed reductions in nuclear arsenals will still leave them capable of destroying the planet many times over. Also, in the enthusiasm for improved East-West relations, the effects of the arms business on developing countries must not be forgotten. All countries with a major involvement in the arms business must be urged to take action, it is not enough to leave it to superpower negotiations. Such action includes:

- reductions in military expenditure, coupled with real progress in negotiations to wind down the nuclear arms race;
- moves toward non-provocative defence policies;
- steps to reduce the international arms trade;
- positive use of the resources freed by the above steps, some of which could certainly be used to provide for improvements in health care;
- investment in the conversion of military industry to socially useful production.

At the root of the arms business, however, are militarism and the reliance of governments on the threat of force to deal with conflict – as highlighted by the proliferation of provocative defence policies. Progress towards disarmament and a more peaceful world requires the political will of governments – and serious steps towards the peaceful resolution of conflict. Certainly strong political will is required if the activities of the arms traders are to be substantially reduced, let alone brought to an end.

The arms business has always insisted, Anthony Sampson notes in *The Arms Bazaar*, that it is like any other business, with no special moral responsibility:

> The involvement of governments has encouraged arms salesmen to delegate any misgivings; but the governments deliberately conceal the full extent and implications of the trade, for fear of arousing public opinion and 'left-wing extremists' . . . the ordinary citizen is right in thinking that the arms trade, like narcotics or slavery, is different from other trades. The more the public is informed and involved, the more prospect there will be of achieving a saner world. (p. 338)

REFERENCES

Alternative Defence Commission, *Without the Bomb: Non-nuclear Defence Policies for Britain* (London, 1985).

M. Brzoska and T. Ohlson, 'The Trade in Major Conventional Weapons', in SIPRI, *World Armaments and Disarmament: SIPRI Yearbook 1986* (Oxford, 1986).

Campaign Against Arms Trade, *Death on Delivery* (London, Campaign Against Arms Trade, 1989).

Campaign Against Arms Trade, *Iran and Iraq: Arms Sales and the Gulf War* (London, Campaign Against Arms Trade factsheet, 1986).

Campaign Against Arms Trade, *Newsletter* (bi-monthly).

G. Hagmeyer-Gaverus, 'World Military Expenditure', in SIPRI, *World Armaments and Disarmament: SIPRI Yearbook 1986* (Oxford, 1986).

T. Ohlson and E. Skons, 'The Trade in Major Conventional Weapons', in SIPRI, *World Armaments and Disarmament: SIPRI Yearbook 1987* (Oxford, 1987).

A. Sampson, *The Arms Bazaar* (London, 1977).

R. Sivard, *World Military & Social Expenditures* (Washington, World Priorities, 1986, 1987-88 and 1989).

US Bureau of Labor Statistics, *The Structure of the US Economy in 1980 and 1985* (Washington, US Bureau of Labor Statistics, 1975).

FURTHER READING

Campaign Against Arms Trade, *Death on Delivery* (London, CAAT, 1989). This booklet examines the impact of the arms trade on the Third World; it explores the nature of the arms trade with the Third World and its links with poverty, debt, war and repression.

Campaign Against Arms Trade, *Newsletter* (bi-monthly). This bi-monthly newsletter focuses on Britain's involvement in the arms trade and contains news of the latest arms contracts plus other developments. It also includes regular features on different aspects of the international arms trade.

R. Sivard, *World Military & Social Expenditures 1989* (Washington, World Priorities, 1989). Published annually, this title provides a useful analysis of the current state of military spending and its social impact. It is packed with invaluable statistics and the country-by-country breakdown covers health, education and nutrition as well as military expenditure.

Third world debt

John Clark and David Keen

> And, in a merry sport,
> If you repay me not on such a day,
> In such a place, such sum or sums as are
> Express'd in the condition, let the forfeit
> Be nominated for an equal pound
> Of your fair flesh, to be cut off and taken
> In what part of your body pleaseth me.
> (Shylock in *The Merchant of Venice*)

In Charles Dickens' day, one baby in six born in Britain died before it

Figure 5.1   Infant mortality in England and Wales

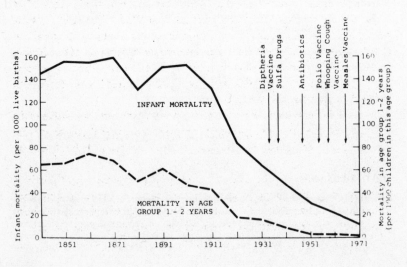

Figure 5.2   Infant mortality in England and Wales

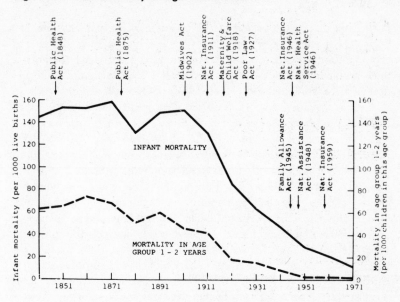

was one year old. Today, the level has dropped to one in sixty. Fig. 5.1 shows that infant mortality in England and Wales was already falling dramatically years before most of the major advances in vaccines and lifesaving drugs. Fig. 5.2 shows that critical items of legislation on health and welfare appear to have had a major impact in reducing infant mortality. In particular, the rush of major welfare reforms before and after the First World War seems to have played a key role in sending infant mortality rates tumbling. Medical advances, then, were less important than tackling the root causes of bad health, such as poor housing and sanitation and lack of income. Tackling poverty proved, in England and Wales, to be the road to better health. Prevention rather than cure was the message.

Because the biggest health hazard has always been poverty, and because the international debt crisis is deepening poverty on a massive scale, those who are concerned about international health must also be concerned about international debt.

Most people in the West have a passing acquaintance with something called the 'debt crisis'; it pops regularly in and out of the news, accompanied by much unfamiliar jargon. Thus international banks are habitually subject to 'exposure', debt payments are repeatedly 'rescheduled', while the IMF is forever imposing its policies of 'adjustment' on debtor countries.

Debt and death

But behind the jargon, behind the TV coverage of international summits, behind the much reported negotiations between international bankers and debtor governments, there is a story that is not so often told. It is the story of those people for whom the 'debt crisis' really is a crisis: a crisis of life and death. For the world's poorest people, debt can be as deadly as drought or war. Vast sums of money move from the less developed countries to the industrialised countries in the form of debt servicing. Because of this drain of funds and the domestic policies imposed by the industrialised countries (through the IMF and the World Bank) to facilitate future repayments, many less developed countries have made drastic cuts in spending on primary health care, education and the relief of poverty. These are precisely areas in which spending has always unlocked the door to improvements in health; any cuts in such spending result in a sharp deterioration in health for large numbers of people.

Government spending cuts are not the only way in which debt can kill. A variety of other policy changes, like too-sudden devaluations, made at the behest of the IMF or the World Bank, have brought widespread increases in hardship and ill-health. The less developed countries are repaying their debts not just with money, but with human lives and human suffering. Yet the industrialised countries have insisted on repayment and austerity as unrelentingly as Shylock demanded his pound of flesh.

In 1989, total Third World debt service stood at $163 billion (roughly half in interest payments and the other half in capital repayments). This was more than three times the amount of total aid contributed by the North. The net transfer of resources from the debt-crisis countries as a whole to developed countries reached $40 billion in 1989 (World Bank). How did so huge a burden of debts and service payments arise? In 1973 oil prices were quadrupled and the major oil-producing states were suddenly acquiring money much faster than they could spend it. They deposited their 'money mountains' in western commercial banks, which then courted the finance ministers of less developed countries so as to obtain new borrowers. The consequent rush of North-to-South lending did not build foundations for prosperity in the borrowing countries.

One large part of the loans was used to pay greatly increased bills for imported oil. Much was also used to finance a boom in prestige projects and imported goods (as in Chile), or to pay for armaments (as in Argentina) and a lot of money that could have funded development vanishes in flights of capital (as from Mexico and the Philippines).

A triple shock for debtors

Much, too, was spent on power stations, airports and capital-intensive industries employing relatively few people. There were few benefits for ordinary people. The disadvantages inherent in such patterns of 'development' were intensified in the late 1970s and early 1980s by a triple shock for the debtors. Oil prices rose again in 1979, increasing the energy costs of the less developed countries that import oil. Interest rates began to rocket in the late 1970s, adding greatly to the burden of repayments for debtor countries, particularly since new loans were often needed to service old loans. The third shock was recession in the industrialised countries. This led to a drop in demand for the commodities of less developed countries at precisely the time when they could least cope with it.

Just a run of bad luck for debtor countries? Not exactly: in many ways, the industrialised countries were simply 'exporting' hardship. Soaring interest rates, for example, largely stemmed from the escalating US budget deficit (around $200 billion at the end of 1987) which was met by US government borrowing. Since most of the budget deficit was incurred to meet US military spending of around $300 billion a year and the rest to keep US taxes down and finance domestic spending, the world's poor were in effect being asked, or rather told, to share the bill for US weaponry. While the US government (and organisations like the IMF in which it plays a leading role) called for austerity and 'good housekeeping' from indebted, less developed countries, it conspicuously failed to follow its own advice when it came to spending in the US.

Even after the succession of shocks hitting debtor countries, crisis was averted so long as *confidence* in their ability to repay their loans was maintained. The international banking community resembled a cartoon figure who runs over the edge of a cliff and yet stays suspended in mid-air – until he looks down and sees the danger he is in. One day in August 1982 the Mexican government called its creditors together to tell them that its current reserves would cover only twelve minutes worth of imports. The banking community was looking into an abyss. Confidence collapsed and the world tumbled into the debt crisis.

Austerity

Debtor countries could not meet their repayments – but the banking community could not afford to write off the debts and further shake the confidence of their investors. Under IMF stewardship the banks reached agreement with their debtors, allowing slower repayments and sometimes lending new money with which they could pay interest. As a condition, debtor governments have been obliged to agree to IMF programmes of adjustment to their economies. The programmes are designed to improve the debtor countries' balance of trade by generating a surplus with which debts can be repaid. Typically, the programmes include government spending cuts, restrictions on domestic credit expansion, and currency devaluation, all tending to reduce imports and inflation and promote the production of goods for export.

The World Bank and the IMF stress the advantages, for debtor countries, of recovery programmes that combine domestic austerity and a boost to exports. Two major problems with this approach have emerged.

First, when many countries attempt simultaneously to expand their exports of a limited range of crops and minerals the supply outstrips the demand and prices for these products tumble. So the approach has proved to be self-defeating and whenever demand has already been reduced by recession and/or the development of substitute products, the fall in price has been especially severe, as with sugar, tin and palm oil prices, to take three examples.

The second problem is that, even where programmes of adjustment might in the long term or even the short term lead to improvements in certain economic indicators (like the balance of trade), the consequences of these programmes for vast numbers of people living in supposedly 're-covering' countries has been grave. Faced with bankers' demands for cuts, governments have had to weigh the likely political consequences of particular types of cuts. Any cuts in city infrastructure, in bloated city-based bureaucracies or in the budgets of modern hospitals and universities, mean running the risk of urban disquiet of the kind that has sometimes brought governments down. Cuts in the armed forces create a risk of insurrection from disgruntled military. The politically easiest way for governments has often been to cut things that directly affect the well-being of poor, and often poorly organised, rural people: primary education, rural health care, agricultural support for small farmers and the like. From them that hath not (and hath not political power), much shall be taken away: the 'trickle down' of poverty (Clark, *For Richer for Poorer*).

Burdens on Jamaica, Zambia, Brazil

An Oxfam report in 1985 showed that 40 per cent of Jamaica's export earnings go to service its debt. After five IMF negotiations since 1977 the government adopted austerity measures that had disastrous effects on poor people (Coote). Price controls and the removal of subsidies were combined with a policy of wage restraint. Basic food prices rose 61 per cent in 1984, by late 1985 a third of the labour force was earning less than £5 per week. As prices outstripped wages, there was a sharp increase in both rural and urban hunger, with the malnutrition rate of under-fives rising to 28 per cent. Unemployment was escalating (to 30 per cent in 1984), fuelled by

than critics and campaigners across the whole sphere of local authority activity.

Their role in improving housing conditions was undermined by a government decision to opt for quantity rather than quality. The Clean Air Act, which significantly reduced inequality in respiratory diseases in the generation now approaching middle age and its successors, stands virtually alone as an example of a new area of health activity by the local authority wing of the NHS in the 1948-74 period.

In the social services, health service and local authority reorganisations of the early 1970s the local authority health departments were split up between the social services departments, the environmental health departments and the community nursing services of the health authorities. Those parts remaining with the local authority ceased to be regarded as part of the NHS. Environmental health departments became the custodians of a set of functions rather than of a social goal. Many authorities transferred the responsibility for housing improvement to their housing departments, breaking a long history of viewing housing policy as a health issue (in 1948 we had a Minister of Health and Housing!). Some authorities added consumer protection to the duties of the environmental health department, apparently in the belief that inspecting things was its main role. Deprived of the leadership of an officer who had a broad advisory responsibility to the council, deprived of its status as part of the NHS, deprived of its links with other health-oriented local authority services, and confined to a limited set of functions, the environmental health departments were relegated to the sidelines.

Reorganisation also destroyed the *post* of medical officer of health although in theory it did not destroy the *role*. This was transferred to the new speciality of community medicine. Although community physicians were to be employed by the NHS, there was a duty laid on health authorities to provide medical advice to local authorities and it was envisaged that the role of the community physician as a local authority officer would continue. In practice the community physician was employed by a different authority, had responsibilities to that authority as well as the council and lacked any executive powers (except in the limited field of communicable disease control) to establish a place in the pecking order. This was a weak position from which to maintain any power in the town hall.

The gap became increasingly obvious and led to the establishment of local authority health units by a number of councils, a development that is discussed in Chapter 10. However, these units also faced the difficulties of being new in a pecking order of power.

These changes in health services are commonly described as a reorganisation and integration of the NHS. They were certainly a reorganisation.

Whether they were an integration is a matter of opinion – they produced a more integrated NHS structure, but only by excluding the bits that did not fit. The services which were originally part of the NHS are no more integrated now than they were before; in fact they became split between four authorities (health, family practitioner committees, social services and environmental health) instead of three. The most important point is that there was a *redefinition*.

The creation of social services departments and the subsequent, but closely linked, reorganisation of the NHS, left outside the NHS the services that followed social or environmental models of health care rather than the medical model. The NHS, thus redefined, was a medical service pure and simple, embodying no other model of health than the medical model, and it was a single bureaucratic structure, whereas before the reorganisation it had not been either of these things.

When the founders of the NHS said that it would reduce inequality in health, they were not necessarily expressing the naïve faith in medical care which is usually read into that statement today – they may have been talking about environmental health. When trade unions in the 1950s and 1960s called for an occupational health service as part of the NHS they probably did not envisage that it would be run by hospital management committees or executive councils and dominated by doctors – they probably envisaged a comprehensive, independently structured service as the fourth wing of the NHS.

There are those who believe that the redefinition should be reversed, and that there is value in the concept of a common identity and sense of common purpose for all the major public agencies through which society pursues health as a social goal. If these people express themselves by saying that social services, environmental health, local authority health units, the Health and Safety Executive and workplace health and safety services should be part of the NHS, they are likely to be misunderstood as advocating a particular medically dominated bureaucratic structure, when in reality this is the reverse of what they mean. In providing us with a term for the bureaucratic entity that is under the direct control of the Secretary of State, the redefinition of the NHS has deprived us of a term for the collectivity of services pursuing health as a social goal. Deprived of a term to express that concept, the concept becomes, as Orwell pointed out, 'literally unthinkable'. This is unfortunate because it is a concept of considerable importance.

Decline in public health activity

In addition to the abolition of the century-old post of medical officer of health, any hopes that the 1974 reorganisation might herald a renaissance of the public health tradition proved sadly misplaced. The NHS offered an inhospitable base both politically and professionally for public health initiatives. Politically, the reluctance of unelected health authorities to criticise other agencies or raise controversial issues of national or local policy restricted the scope for forthright advocacy on public health. Professionally, the public health doctors had weakened their institutional links with areas like environmental health, social services and housing, and gained instead a base in which the major emphasis lay on providing treatment services. Lacking support for significant innovations in public health, and further hampered by recruitment difficulties following successive rounds of retirements, community medicine specialists often became bogged down in a heterogeneous collection of management tasks like organising school health services and health education. Their role as medical advisers to health authorities also landed them with an ill-defined negotiating role among powerful internal interest groups over which they had no direct control. Although the 1982 reorganisation of the NHS simplified the cumbersome structures established in 1974, it made no attempt to clarify or strengthen the public health role of the service.

When the changes to the organisation of the NHS emerging from the inquiry headed by Sir Roy Griffiths were introduced in 1985, the marginal status of the public health doctors made them extremely vulnerable, since in many districts they were seen as neither practising clinicians nor trained managers. Although the DHSS sought to square the circle with a semantic distinction between 'professional accountability' to the health authority and 'managerial accountability' to the general manager, in reality there was often very little room for additional senior (and expensive) posts between the already powerful clinicians and the newly powerful general managers. The establishment by the DHSS in 1986 of the Acheson Inquiry into the future of public health and community medicine represented a belated recognition of the crisis of identity facing the public health doctors (Harvey and Judge).

The Acheson Inquiry prompted some extravagant claims about the role and potential of community medicine. Not surprisingly, the Faculty of Community Medicine offered the most comprehensive view, arguing for a leading role for community physicians in epidemiology, health service planning, health promotion and the prevention of disease, collaboration with local authorities, advising the public on health issues, medical manpower planning, and professional communication with other medical bodies such as family practitioner committees. The Faculty of Community Medicine drew quite explicitly on the historical tradition of the medical officers of health at a number of points – notably in arguing for a return to the publication of annual reports and for the need for community physicians to enjoy 'a more secure tenure of appointment . . . than has prevailed since the early 1970s in order to allow them to speak publicly where necessary on "politically sensitive" issues'.

Considering the enthusiasm with which the public health doctors pursued NHS integration in 1974, there is no small irony in the attempt to recreate elements of their local authority past. More generally, it could be argued that the need to establish the Acheson Inquiry in the first place arose only because the practice of community medicine at least since 1974 bore only limited resemblance to the roles claimed by the faculty. Certainly, examples of high-calibre contributions in all these areas could be identified, just as there were examples of continued commitment to broad public health approaches by individual medical officers right up to 1974 (Godber). But in many districts there was a marked absence of accessible epidemiological data on which to base policy decisions; collaboration with other agencies was often patchy and at worst chaotic; and health promotion remained under-resourced and marginal.

Clearly these failings could not be blamed solely on community medicine; for example, the absence of any coherent strategies for primary care services or community care owed more to government policy decisions than to local inadequacies. But even when due allowance is made for the difficulties under which they laboured, the limited professional, political and public impact made by the relocated public health doctors is striking. For example, the publication of the Black Report in 1980 offered an excellent opportunity both to undertake parallel epidemiological investigations on a local basis and to highlight the national and local implications of the report's broad-ranging recommendations on issues of traditional public health concern such as housing, poverty and occupational health. With some honourable exceptions, community physicians shied away from such responses; indeed, even where local work on deprivation and ill-health was undertaken, it was often done as part of a narrow argument about the allocation of resources within the NHS, rather than as a broader attempt to rebuild a political and professional constituency for public health interventions. Similarly, within the NHS, the imposition of privatisation involved redundancies and reductions in the wages, holidays, sick pay, maternity rights and pension rights of precisely those staff whose health status was already the most deprived. Although the public health implications of such policies were clear, few community physicians were willing to intervene publicly on this 'politically sensitive issue' by forcing their health authorities to acknowledge the health consequences of their actions.

Such criticisms of community medicine in no way absolve other agencies – notably local authorities – from their share of responsibility for the decline in public health activity. However, in a whole range of areas, it is the historic role of public health doctors, already reduced, that is being still further contested. Thus GPs and paediatricians jostle for primacy in child health services; environmental health officers resist presumptions of medical leadership in control of communicable diseases; health education officers, like social workers and environmental health officers before them, grow increasingly restive under medical domination; and local authority responses to Acheson have emphasised that specifically medical advice is only one element in the formulation of public health policies. Given the range and complexity of the contemporary public health task, it is hardly surprising that a century-old structure should have been found wanting. But the creation of new structures that will be as relevant to the problems of the future as the medical officer of health was to the problems of the past remains an urgent need.

Medical organisations

The BMA has a long history of public health campaigning, perhaps best exemplified recently by its campaigns against the tobacco industry, boxing and alcohol and its campaigns for road safety. Although the public is often surprised by the forthrightness of these campaigns, especially from a body generally seen as part of the establishment, they actually derive from very deep roots. The BMA has engaged in public health campaigns virtually from its foundation. In the nineteenth century it made statements about social conditions, including housing, industrial legislation, and the Poor Law, that placed it unequivocally on the side of social reform.

These traditions run contrary, however, to another powerful tradition of medicine, the concept of medicine as non-political. This tradition is particularly powerful because it protects the legitimacy of a medical opinion, almost universally accepted unquestioningly as unbiased. The two traditions are least in conflict where a campaign, although controversial, and perhaps involving conflict with powerful vested interests or deeply held political assumptions, is not party-political. In that situation the BMA will give priority to its public health traditions and place itself at the forefront of a campaign. Thus the BMA is not afraid to confront the power of the tobacco lobby, for smoking is not a party issue or a Left/Right issue, and the tobacco industry may be separated out as evil and untypical of industry as a whole, so the issue raises no fundamental anti-capitalist stance. Similarly the BMA was prepared, over the issue of seat-belt legislation, to confront the powerful libertarian assumptions of British politics, for to do so again entailed no party-political stance – Margaret Thatcher and Michael Foot stood together in opposition to the legislation.

It is where public health has a party-political element or seems to strike at the roots of social organisation that the issue will be more complex. In these situations fierce debates will take place between those who place the priority on the need to campaign for health and those who argue that the BMA should take no political stance. Examples of such debates can be seen in the controversy that surrounded its reports on nuclear war and on deprivation and health.

The same general attitude is taken by most of the main medical organisations, with the obvious exception of the Medical Practitioners Union which, as the medical organisation of the Labour movement, tends to be much more willing to draw political conclusions about health. This often makes its position more controversial than the view of a more broadly based organisation. It is tempting to argue that medical bodies should change to explicit socio-political criticism. Yet the 'non-political' nature of the medical profession does enhance a medical opinion and changing it might prove counter-productive. Organisations like the Medical Practitioners Union, as well as the radical community physicians, also benefit from the 'non-political' mantle cast over the profession. If the profession were seen as Left-wing and anti-capitalist the whole of the BMA's public health campaigning would be undermined. It would, however, be valuable if a medical campaign for public health were to be started on a broader base than the Medical Practitioners Union, but with a less cautious attitude to politics than that taken by the main organisations in medicine. Such an organisation might be either an independent association or a medical section of the Public Health Alliance.

REFERENCES

Faculty of Community Medicine, *The Role and Function of the Specialty of Community Medicine* (London, Faculty of Community Medicine, 1986).
G.E. Godber, 'Medical Officers of Health and Health Services', *Community Medicine*, 8, 1 (1986).
S. Harvey and K. Judge, *Community Medicine and the NHS in England* (London, Kings Fund Institute, 1988).
C. Webster, 'Medical Officers of Health – for the Record', *Radical Community Medicine*, Autumn 1986.
A.S. Wohl, *Endangered Lives: Public Health in Victorian Britain* (London, 1983).

FURTHER READING

J. Lewis, *What Price Community Medicine. The Philosophy, Practice and Politics of Public Health since 1919* (Brighton, 1986). A useful review of the development of community medicine as a specialty and of the problems which prompted the establishment of the Acheson Inquiry.
Unit for the Study of Health Policy, *Rethinking Community Medicine* (London, Guys Hospital Medical School, 1979). A cogent argument for the development of a broad-

based contemporary public health movement, and for the potential of community medicine specialists to collaborate in this development rather than becoming bogged down in the managerial and administrative minutiae of the NHS.

The articles by Godber and Webster (see References) offer sharply contrasting views of the contributions made by medical officers of health both before and after the introduction of the NHS.

A.S. Wohl, *Endangered Lives: Public Health in Victorian Britain* (London, 1983). A review of the whole range of public health issues facing the Victorians, and of the political and economic context within which these were addressed, both nationally and locally. Extensive bibliography.

Environmental health officers
Peter Allen

Who are our local 'environmental' watchdogs?

In one sense the whole local community has an 'environmental' watchdog responsibility. The most effective action takes place when a community, or part of a community, identifies a particular issue, be it noise, pollution from a factory or unhygienic food handling at a local restaurant. However, within this framework the development of modern public health since the nineteenth century has shown that a professional input is necessary for these and similar issues to be properly dealt with. Different professionals are involved with local environmental issues, not least the environmental health officer. But where are these to be found and what can they do?

Where are environmental health officers to be found?

Following the Local Government Act of 1974, which modernised local government, broadly three types of local authorities have emerged. The County Councils, which are concerned with issues such as education, social services and trading standards and which cover the large geographical county areas; the local District Councils, whose responsibilities include housing, recreation and environmental health; and the Metropolitan District Councils, which are centred on large areas of population like Leeds and Birmingham, and combine the functions of both District and County Councils. The London Boroughs were also modernised in the 1970s and like the Metropolitan District Councils, combine both District and County functions.

Although some environmental health officers are employed by County Councils, and indeed by private companies and government departments,

Figure 6.1   A modern environmental health department

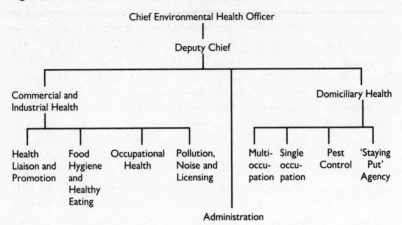

most are employed by local councils – the District Councils, the Metropolitan Districts and thhe London Boroughs. Therefore it is through the door of the local council offices that one must go to find the local environmental health department.

The above figure illustrates the arrangement of a modern environmental health department. Before considering the contribution that it can make to advancing a positive public health policy, it is worth looking at the powers of environmental health officers and the limitations of these powers.

Pollution and noise

Under the Public Health Act and the Environmental Protection Act 1990 the officer has fairly extensive powers to monitor and, in defined cases, to intervene legally. Smoke, odours, noise, noxious gases, dust and radioactivity can all be addressed.

However, there are important legal limitations, especially where industry and commerce are concerned. If a local council wishes, for instance, to take action against a local factory for allowing paint to be emitted on nearby residents, it must prove not only that this fallout causes a nuisance, but that the company is not taking the best practicable means to prevent the nuisance. This sounds simple enough until the law is tested in court. Not only does the environmental health officer have to prove that the paint is coming from a particular factory, but also that it is affecting people directly (landing on their property is not enough). The officer must go on to show that 'best practicable means' has not been taken, and here the cost of putting the situation right as well as the feasibility of the technology have to be taken into consideration. For a large factory the cost could amount to millions of pounds, which the company would probably argue was prohibitive. Finally, even if the action is successful, the maximum fine can be derisory. See, for instance, Oxford City Council v British Leyland. The fine was a mere £1,000. The Environmental Protection Act of 1990 brought some improvements, but problems can be expected in defining 'excessive costs' and the contents of the guidance notes.

Often no action can be taken until after an offence has been committed. A farmer can set up a huge rearing area for, say, pheasants or poultry in a field at the back of a private house. The fact that similar establishments in other places have given rise to smell, noise and fly nuisances does not enable the health officer to prevent the problem arising. The 'out of bounds' limitation is another problem. This affects water, nuclear power stations and 'scheduled' processes. The local authority's health officers can monitor the state of the water under the new Water Act, but they do not have the power to prosecute. The government has given that power to two non-elected, centrally constituted bodies, the National Rivers Authority and the National Drinking Water Inspectorate. Environmental health officers can also monitor radioactivity, but again cannot prosecute. Similarly the government has designated certain 'scheduled' processes within factories to be 'out of bounds' and reserved the right to regulate these through a centralised inspectorate. Central inspectorates have a role to play, but too often they are thin on the ground, lack local accountability and are not around when the problem occurs.

So, although the environmental health department does have a number of powers, in important aspects those powers are inadequate to resolve the public health problems of the 1990s.

Food hygiene and healthy eating

Another traditional role of the environmental health officer has been in food hygiene. Under the Food Acts and Food Hygiene Regulations, the officer can inspect food premises and prosecute where these infringe the statute, and also has powers in relation to food poisoning and food handling. The officers, with other concerned groups, have been exercising their watchdog role during the 1980s by 'barking' about the inadequacies of the present food hygiene legislation. This includes allowing food premises to be opened without clearance to ensure that the operation is hygienic and safe; the lack of any requirement that managers or employees involved in food handling should have even a smattering of food hygiene knowledge; the fact that certain government establishments can hide behind 'crown immunity' and so avoid prosecution; and the pitiful penalties.

Following the food scares of the 1980s involving salmonella, listeria, BST and BSE and so on, the government has committed itself to remedy some of the deficiencies by legislation. However, in terms of developing a positive public health policy, the question must be asked: why do people have to suffer illness or die before there is a will to change the law? How much barking does a watchdog have to do before it is heard?

Occupational health

Traditionally the health and safety of factory employees have been 'watch-dogged' by factory inspectors (now health and safety inspectors). Since the Health and Safety Act of 1974 common standards are now, broadly speaking, applied to all offices, shops and factories where people are employed. The administration of the Act is shared between the government's inspectors and the local authority's environmental health officers. At times this can be confusing, not only to the public but also to the enforcement officers themselves. However, the local authority's officers enforce the Act mainly in the retail and distribution sector. In the year 1987/88, 989,000 premises fell within the ambit of the local authorities and 528,000 visits were made. Comparable health and safety sector figures showed 700,000 premises within the province of government inspectors and 173,033 visits made.

Whilst acknowledging the expertise of the government's specialist inspectors, it seems not just confusing but puzzling that, at the local level, we need two sets of 'generic' officers, one with accountability to the local community, the other without. In developing a positive public health policy this issue would need to be examined.

Domiciliary health

Environmental health officers have traditionally been involved in the battle against poor housing. Today that battle seems more of a rearguard action. The government's latest House Condition Survey (1987), carried out by seconded health officers and other surveyors, shows that 4.8 per cent of the total housing stock is 'unfit'. That does not sound too bad until one begins to define 'unfit'. According to the statutory definition of unfitness, which harks back to the nineteenth century, a house can lack an inside WC and a hot water supply, be in grave disrepair and thoroughly damp, yet still fall outside the 'unfit' category. The statutory definition shrouds the true state of our housing stock.

Today a generally accepted standard of fitness which takes into consideration such matters as basic amenities, the state of repair, and adequate roof insulation, is found in the '10 point improvement grant' standard. In a 1,000 house survey carried out in Oxford at the same time as the government's survey, it was found that only 57.7 per cent of houses met that standard. If that is the situation in what many would judge a fairly affluent southern city, what must it be like in less privileged areas!

We cannot have a positive public health policy which allows our housing to fall into disrepair.

I am not going to comment on pest control, because I am sure most readers of this book will realise the importance of such a service and will be aware of the need to keep vigilant. However, the 'Staying Put' Agency in figure 6.1 perhaps needs comment. One area of housing which is particularly bad is that occupied by retired people. Cash problems, fear of being ripped off by unscrupulous builders and a general feeling that to organise a repair job is all too much, have led many retired people to neglect the fabric of their homes. Therefore, an increasing number of environmental health departments are setting up – alone or with a Housing Association – a 'one stop service'. This enables a retired person to hand over the problem of getting work done to the agency. The agency arranges the work, chooses the builder and locates grants if these are applicable. Those who can afford to pay are charged a small commission. The initiative, commendable as it is, will not be sufficient unless more resources are provided.

General

Health promotion

An environmental health practitioner will mainly be involved with the environmental aspects of health promotion, but can also be in a good position to carry out activities that advance personal and social health. For instance, officers hopefully will ensure that food premises and practices within their area are kept up to a good standard. Their primary aim in doing this is to advance health environmentally. However, one result of these activities will be fewer cases of food poisoning, so they are also advancing personal and social health. An increasing number of environmental health departments are participating in the Health Education Authority's 'Heartbeat' award scheme, which extends this contribution to advancing personal and social health by encouraging the provision of healthy-choice menus and no-smoking areas. Some environmental health departments are going even further and are initiating and facilitating strategies designed primarily towards personal and social health advance. We only have to look at the pioneering work carried out by environmental health departments in the fields of AIDS, smoking and alcohol consumption to find evidence of this.

So, although environmental health officers are primarily interested in health promotion as it affects the environment, they will have opportunities to use their skill and knowledge to make contributions in the other fields of health.

Cost

The District Auditor's figures for 1986 show that the average expenditure per head of population in England and Wales on environmental health (including health promotion) was £8 per year or just over 15 pence per week. The average cost of keeping a pet dog in canned dog food, not to mention the vet's fees, is £3.50 per week! In developing a positive public health policy we have to ask whether we have got our priorities right.

What can environmental health officers contribute to advancing a positive public health policy?

So much for the powers and limitations of an environmental health department. What is perhaps of more importance is the specific contribution that its officers can make to advancing a positive public health policy, both in concept and in practice. Clearly the type of contribution will vary from one local authority to another, depending on local circumstances such as the needs of the area, the vision of the elected members, the resources available and, of course, the 'personalities' of local participants. Nevertheless, it is suggested that there are five main ways in which an environmental health officer can help:

(1) Personal and social health and well-being is determined in no small measure by the quality of the environment and from our previous section it can be seen that officers have the capacity, given the resources, to make a substantial direct contribution to the health of the community in such areas as occupational health, food hygiene and pollution control.

(2) Moreover, because of their traditional links with the former medical officer of health, now the director of public health medicine, the environmental health officers are in a good position to encourage the health authority to play a greater preventive role in the local community.

(3) Environmental health officers provide what is essentially a local government delivery service. This brings them into a close working relationship not only with the local community, but with local commerce,

local industry and local voluntary organisations and so on. They are therefore in a useful position to advance health within these networks.

(4) Environmental health departments are also the local authority's 'health headquarters', often with their own chief officer. So staff are in a unique position to encourage other local authority departments such as recreation and personnel to look at their health contributions. This point is expanded in Chapter 10.

(5) Last, but by no means least, the officers can make a significant contribution to public health policy via their own professional network. Britain has about 6,500 practising environmental health officers. This provides a network that is small enough for effective communication to take place. This was illustrated in Oxford in 1987 when we held a Healthy City Exchange. Twenty key cities responded to our invitation to exchange ideas and working examples of health initiatives.

Environmental health officers in perspective

Finally, we turn to two questions: when did the environmental health officers first take on a watchdog role and what sort of role can they expect in the future?

The past, and perhaps the future, can be best seen within the context of the development of public health generally. This development falls into four periods, each period characterised by a special emphasis.

From the 1830s to the 1880s, there was, prompted by the ravages of infectious diseases which swept across the land, intervention about sanitation, at the very basic level of providing clean water and a reasonable sewerage system, plus occasional forays into bad housing and bad food. It was during this phase that the environmental health officer came into being. The legislative midwife was the Public Health Act, 1848, which established the office of Inspector of Nuisances. After a name change to Sanitary Inspector and another to Public Health Inspector, the title was finally changed to Environmental Health Officer.

From 1880 to 1930 there was intervention at the personal and social level, fueled by the horrendous results of medical examinations of recruits for the Boer War, many of whom had to be turned down as unfit for service. The school meals, school medical, health visitor, district nursing and midwifery services were all established in this period. Environmental health work developed during this period, as is shown by the medical officer of health's annual reports in which the chief sanitary inspector would often have his own section, as for instance, Thomas Hull in the Oxford reports. The high profile development was not at District Council level, however, but at the new County Council level where the personal and social health services began to make themselves felt.

From 1930-1970, following Alexander Fleming's antibiotic discovery and the other drug breakthroughs of this time, came the therapeutic intervention period, with vaccines, vitamins and contraceptives having a profound effect on public health. Public health workers were also still busy tackling such matters as the huge slum clearance programme, getting to grips with food poisoning and unhygienic food premises and beginning to look at the ill-health caused by insanitary offices and shops.

However, from the 1970s, public health in the UK and elsewhere has been characterised by a totally new type of approach – the holistic one. This recognises that all factors need to be considered if our communities are to have positive health, including such matters as poverty, the economic framework, inequalities and so forth. The corollary is that no single organisation or profession has all the answers; that if the goal of positive public health is to be attained, there is a need to welcome inputs from all directions, not least from the community itself.

The future

So where do environmental health officers fit into this fourth, critical, phase? Well, I suggest that they, as the 'health professionals' within the elected local authority, are in a good position to help open up the local authority and community to other professions and other organisations and similarly to open up other professions and organisations to the local community.

At present the signs are not encouraging. Structural factors mentioned elsewhere in this book tend to be moving the scene of activity away from local government and thus away from local accountability. Where major public health problems are revealed, governments find it expedient to adopt a quick 'centralised' policy. This is not to say that central action is not needed, but rather that there is a need for a pluralistic approach which encourages and provides for both central and local action.

Local government is in danger of being marginalised and with this will go local accountability. Without local accountability it is all too easy, when public outcry and agitation have turned to other things, for resources to be reduced or switched elsewhere. In 1976 the Royal Commission on Environmental Pollution reviewed air pollution. It called for the number of inspectors dealing with air pollution centrally to be doubled. Then there were forty-seven, now, at the time of writing, there are thirty-two. Similarly with the government's factory inspectors – these reached an all time 'high' of 759 in 1980 (a pathetically low figure when you consider the size of their workload). In 1988 this number was down to 592. Local accountability is needed to keep the pressure up while the problems remain.

In addition, local authorities themselves have been, and are being, squeezed. Privatisation of services means less scope to meet public health needs. For example, the privatisation of council housing, coupled with controls on new buildings, has been accompanied by an increase in homelessness – the market has not provided! Local authority finance is also facing an incredibly difficult future. Whether we call it the community charge or the poll tax the net result is the same: less cash for local authorities and for public health initiatives.

Since the environmental health department is an integral part of the local authority, it will be directly affected by these changes and will have less freedom to act. The fact that there is an acute shortage of staff (officially recognised by both government and opposition) will further exacerbate the situation. The key issue for a public health policy is whether the monumental problems can force public health back to the top of the agenda.

Watchdog postscript

As we seek to advance a positive public health policy, it's worth remembering that we can learn from history. Not least from the Saxon period. The Saxon villages that dotted the countryside were to a great degree self-reliant and self-governing. Interestingly enough they also had watchdogs: the real thing, shaggy black dogs of wolfish origin. They not only hunted with the community, but at night kept predators at bay by bark, bite or full confrontation. But the important thing was that the watchdogs were an integral part of the Saxon settlement. Modern environmental watchdogs will only be effective if they are part of a community that takes responsibility for its health and in particular for ensuring a sufficient number of properly trained and responsive environmental watchdogs.

REFERENCES

Health and Safety Executive, *Accidents in Service Industries* (London, 1989).
P.F. Allen, 'A Blueprint for Health Advancement', *Health and Hygiene*, 10 (1989).
C.F. Brockington, *A Short History of Public Health* (London, 1966).

CHAPTER 7

Politics and hostile environments

Peter Draper and Stanley Harrison

In this first of three chapters discussing the effects of social conflicts on progress in public health, three kinds of friend are recognised: allies, supporters and watchdogs. Two classic but still relevant battles are analysed. The first is Ralph Nader's indictment in the 1950s of the US automobile industry as a killer; the second is the long war with the world tobacco trade. In different ways each exposed the pitiless philosophy and practices sometimes employed in trade and industry, which sabotage people's health.

The parts played by bureaucratic inertia and inadequate information are also discussed. A broadside is fired at the British parliament's current failure to meet the political needs of the time, with public health as one of the casualties.

Public health as a battleground

Progress in public health has often been achieved by winning battles with the makers or distributors of harmful products. The military metaphor is no mere cliché, it fits the case only too well. We are not all on the same side and the 'war' over our health is a ceaseless and complex affair of advances and setbacks. In the field there are friends and enemies, allies and supporters – and also referees whose whistles are often disobeyed or blown too feebly or too late. Real motives of invading forces are usually hidden and extensive camouflage is in constant use. There are many deliberate diversions, obstacles and traps.

The idea that public health often involves battles is not difficult to understand if one considers, for example, the battles in most countries with the various producers and distributors of hard drugs. These days it is also easy to see those people and institutions still involved in actively promoting the use of tobacco as enemies of public health. Some people and some powerful institutions act in ways that seriously jeopardise people's health, whatever they say about their aims and activities or about public health and it is no accident that the great fictional hero of public health was characterised ironically as 'an enemy of the people'.

Three kinds of friends

Allies

Medical organisations like the BMA often engage in public health battles about major health problems such as smoking or drinking-and-driving, but they try hard to avoid battles that are likely to run along party-political lines. Nursing organisations such as the Royal College of Nursing and the Health Visitors' Association, and health service trade unions like COHSE and NUPE, are other allies from the ranks of people who work in health care. When a specific battleground is identified, there are normally many other allies if their potential is recognised and mobilised through good liaison, literature and videos which arm them with relevant facts and illustrations.

In conflicts about nutrition, the allies range from health educators and teachers to the staff of wholefood shops and restaurants. In the middle are all the various salespeople and producers from greengrocers and people who grow fruit and vegetables in back gardens and on allotments to people who bring out gardening magazines. Similarly, in the promotion of regular physical exercise, the allies range from health educators and PE teachers to the makers of sports equipment, staff and councillors of local recreation and leisure departments, members of sports clubs and associations from rugby to skateboarding. These various groups are certainly not battling away all the time, but they can normally be relied on in an important conflict if they are contacted and armed with campaigning information.

Supporters

Whereas allies of public health are to be found on the battlefields, supporters do not themselves engage in direct combat but they provide ammunition and other vital resources. Critically important are the people and organisations who finance research. This is particularly so in periods when publicly-funded research into sensitive topics is eroded in favour of the interests of powerful groups, such as those who control the brewing industries. All the different kinds of bodies that fund research into the health or environmental impacts of economic or other developments are essential supporters. So are people who disseminate those research findings – from school teachers to broadcasters. Another group of supporters related both to the research and the educational group is what might be called the 'healthy policy and practice people'. They foster the development of healthy public policies such as agricultural policies that help farmers and horticulturists to uncouple themselves from the agrochemical giants, safeguard soil fertility and work in ways that are healthy for farmworkers as well as consumers and neighbours – including all who drink the local water.

Absolutely and relatively, Britain is extremely short of detailed work on the development of policies that make sense in terms of resources, pollution and other factors important to health. There is no evidence that this gap exists because we do not have suitable people. It exists because government funding is mean and short-sighted and because the foundations, industry and government choose to use their research funds for other purposes. Only a few years ago a senior officer at the DHSS reacted to criticism by telling me that his department could look at ecologically sound policies only if they could be disguised as contingency plans.

Since battles for public health are often for real rather than nominal accountability, groups that promote the general cause of public accountability are certainly numbered in the ranks of supporters. Such supporters would include all who favour the defence and improvement of local government rather than the ever-increasing centralisation and distancing of decision-making. They would also include people and groups within the NHS that promote accountability to public and staff, as many Community Health Councils do. Teachers, academics and journalists of all kinds who help people to develop an informed and critical understanding of democracy and policies also contribute indirectly to public health. Also included would be MPs who seek to strengthen parliament and resist Downing Street and Whitehall takeovers of public business. Serving the same kinds of purposes, organisations like Charter 88 also rank as valuable general supporters in pressing for proportional representation and a democratic, non-hereditary second chamber.

Watchdogs

The third kind of friend can bite as well as bark – at least in theory. In the brief histories of medical officers of health and environmental health officers in Chapter 6 we saw, however, that bark and bite can sometimes disappoint. The fundamental problem is often, as now in Britain, that the watchdogs are too few and some are underfed – they lack adequate technical support and are often underpaid. We have noted, for instance, the staff shortages in pollution control and health and safety at work. There can be other power or political problems with watchdogs that we shall return to shortly, though it is salutary to begin by recalling that in extreme cases, like Karen Silkwood and the Greenpeace worker who was blown up by the French secret service, watchdogs are killed by those with something to hide.

In addition to readily identified watchdogs, there are many others who directly and indirectly make a significant contribution to public health. For example, different kinds of community workers commonly make a fuss about poverty and other health-threatening circumstances, including appalling socio-economic conditions which are not understood outside the local communities affected, unhappily far from a rare situation. Other watchdogs of this kind include many GPs, health visitors, social workers, district nurses, the clergy and voluntary workers. School inspectors, too, sometimes draw attention to conditions that jeopardise children's health.

In the voluntary field, watchdogs like Shelter and the Child Poverty Action Group and similar organisations have combined reforming zeal with a painstaking projection of data on social evils that are tolerated partly because of a pervasive ignorance about them. They have come to arch over the national scene with support from a wide public and some footholds in official institutions. With no great victories to celebrate they have nonetheless helped to keep a social conscience alive.

Shelter's housing rights campaign, for instance, in 1987 – the year the United Nations designated the Year of Shelter for the Homeless – aimed to increase public awareness of the ugly facts of housing in Britain and to mobilise the will to tackle them.

The Child Poverty Action Group, which led the campaign at the end of the 1970s to introduce child benefit, has been at war with poverty for over twenty years. It plays a vital role in documenting poverty in Britain. The case it presents, in its journal *Poverty*, in its research reports and surveys, rests on the fact that about nine million people in Britain live on or below the poverty line and two million of them are children. The group fights for increased benefits for the long-term unemployed and the poorest families; and, as it says, it helps to set the agenda for the debate on longer-term reform, and to 'put the security back into Social Security'. When Norman Fowler was Social Services Secretary he said: 'I pay tribute to CPAG and other pressure groups that have formidable expertise'.

The watch kept by these and similar bodies cannot achieve anything other than to inform the public, appeal to its sense of justice or its emotions and evoke active responses. For the watchdogs who are paid employees, a different kind of problem arises when their owners take no notice of their barking and may, indeed, muzzle and attack the dogs before cutting their rations. The plight of environmental protection staff in the US during the Reagan administrations became internationally notorious.

As we saw in Chapter 6, tampering with official statistics is a comparable sin – modulating the bark until it is unrecognisable. Mrs Thatcher's administrations changed the basis of unemployment figures more than thirty times, each of which alterations, surprise, surprise, reduced the official totals. The statistics of poverty were too big to be massaged into a downward trend. One ploy has been to delay the publication of embarrassing figures, sometimes for several years. Another has been to make the publication as inconspicuous as possible – like the time the latest poverty figures were placed in the library of the Commons on the day the House went into recession. Other examples were discussed in Chapter 6.

Professional statisticians are key actors, as we saw briefly in the previous chapter. The scandal of tampering with official statistics peaked in Britain in October 1989 when the Royal Statistical Society decided to consider a proposal for an independent watchdog over the integrity of statistics. The former presidents of the Government Statistical Service and the Royal Statistical Society both traced the decline in standards to a 1981 White Paper entitled 'Government Statistical Services':

> In two and a half pages there were seven references to efficiency, five to value for money, four to economics and two each to savings and cost effectiveness. Integrity, validity and reliability merited one mention each and objectivity got two. (*The Independent*, 9 October 1989)

Sir David Cox commented 'Informed public discussion of potentially controversial issues is being inhibited'. Sir Claus Moser said his main worry 'was about the unemployment statistics, the poverty data and any suggestions of tampering with the Retail Price Index'. He had wanted a national statistics council as a protective agency ten years ago. This revolt of the statisticians themselves followed an earlier book, *Facing the Figures*, from the Radical Statistics Group, and a TV documentary accusing the government of 'cooking the books' over unemployment, poverty and the health service.

Enemies of health

We may usefully start our closer look at the enemy host by recalling a well-documented US confrontation in the health and safety war, because it remains a classic exposure of the ruthless methods used by some corporate giants to sell dangerous products. This was Ralph Nader's indictment of the American automobile industry as a mass killer in the 1950s.

For decades the industry conned drivers into believing that they were going around in marvels of technological efficiency and safety. Nader's demonstration in *Unsafe at Any Speed* (1965) that millions of the 'marvels' were in fact death traps, only inspired General Motors to campaign for years to shift the blame to everything but the design and engineering of the vehicles. A later edition of the book (1973) noted that the monopoly power of General Motors was able to bring to heel even so large a company as Ford when it started a brief flirtation with car safety features like seat-belts and padding for instrument panels as a selling line for a new model. Nader records:

> A classic opportunity for the competitive forces in the marketplace to launch a safety turnabout in the auto industry was crushed by one corporate giant who not only could not stand competition of this kind but was powerful enough to stop it with a few well-placed telephone calls . . . For decades the conventional explanation preferred by the traffic safety establishments and insinuated into the laws, with the backing of the industry and its allies, was that most accidents are caused by wayward drivers who *ipso facto* cause most injuries and deaths. (Nader, 1973)

He described the pitiless pressures and refined trickery, suppression of safety data established by the firms' own engineering research and constant wirepulling whereby the main culprit for the mayhem on the highways was kept shrouded in secrecy. In the six years after the first publication of the book, 330,000 people died in the US as a result of road accidents and twenty-five million more were injured.

The conspiracy – it was no less – revealed the complexity of such conflicts, which are wars of movement rather than battles from static positions of demonstrable right and wrong. It indicated that they are soluble only by wide coalitions of interests able to generate enough political energy to secure change. It took years of in-depth publicity and campaigning, lobbying and electioneering and debate inside and outside the official and business institutions to dispel the American auto industry's myths and pretences and force it to start accepting responsibility for people's safety as users of its products.

Nader's enemies, like enemies of public health in other conflicts, did not of course announce their true aims or motives; nearly always the opponents loudly protest their innocence and are quick to send libel writs against alleged maligners of their integrity. To take an extreme but important example, the various producers and distributors of hard drugs normally maintain silence in public. In no way do they identify themselves as saboteurs of people's health. But the same is usually true, for instance, of serious polluters of land, air or water. Reticence in acknowledging their anti-social role sometimes occurs because they are unwitting offenders, but there are many examples of innocence being adopted as a public relations posture. The tobacco industry provides many cases.

Smokescreens

The tobacco industry has been and remains one of the most fertile sources of protestations of virtue in the teeth of masses of evidence, though it is only in the last few years that well-documented studies of the industry's duplicity have been readily available. In *Smoke Ring: The Politics of Tobacco*, Peter Taylor instances many gaps between the public statements of the tobacco transnationals and their behaviour. In the course of his description of how President Carter's Secretary for Health, Education and Welfare, Joe Califano, was removed from his post because he was too keen to reduce smoking, we learn that – despite the industry's frequent claims that it does not target advertising at children – $2 million meant to inform school-children about the dangers of smoking was removed from his budget. Taylor reports Califano as saying: 'The industry really lobbied to knock that out of the budget . . . It confirmed my suspicions – and now I know – that they really go after the kids: that's who they are after in their advertising; and that's who they're after in trying to sell cigarettes' (p. 215). The BMA, in its *Cigarette Advertising and Smoking* says baldly, 'children are the future of the tobacco industry and therefore primary targets for tobacco advertising. There is ample evidence of their interest in, and recall of, tobacco advertising' (Chapman).

The BBC's science correspondent, James Wilkinson, in his *Tobacco; The Facts Behind the Smokescreen* also documents many cases of the industry sabotaging public health while protesting the opposite. Explaining the tactic of weakening health education on the dangers of smoking by suggesting that the indictment of tobacco is 'unproven' he comments:

From the first moment that cigarettes were linked with illness and especially lung cancer the cigarette manufacturers realised that were they ever to admit that the product they were promoting and selling at huge profit was dangerous, they would open the door to successful product-liability suits. From that moment their stock answer . . . has always been that the link between cigarettes and ill health is unproven. They often add that no one has ever been able to show exactly what is the causal mechanism. This is just a ruse to persuade the gullible that you need to know the exact mechanism to explain *how* something is dangerous before you can say that it *is* dangerous. This is illogical. You do not need to know how antibiotics work, for instance, to realise that they do. (p. 90)

Satisfaction with the considerable success of anti-tobacco campaigns in some developed countries has been diluted by the knowledge that great billows of lethal smoke are simply being blown away from the economic North onto the South. The US cigarette companies, like other tobacco transnationals, have always promoted world sales aggressively and this tendency has strengthened as American domestic demand declined. Today about a third of US males are smokers compared with 52.4 per cent in 1965 (Office on Smoking and Health).

During the past year the US Trade Office has successfully used the threat of trade sanctions to open up and transform the cigarette markets of Japan, Taiwan and South Korea. The changes will greatly encourage the use of milder, easier to inhale tobacco and greatly expand western style cigarette advertising . . . Following patterns in America, the demand for cigarettes could increase particularly among females and adolescents who are currently minimal smokers . . . Westernised cigarette advertising and competition will help spread the smoking epidemic throughout the Far East and the biggest loser could be China. Smoking is relatively new in China with cigarette production rising 500 per cent since 1960 . . . According to British epidemiologist Richard Peto approximately 30,000 lung cancers occurred in 1986 but this should rise to 900,000 annually by 2025. Of the 200 million Chinese children alive today, 50 million will die from smoking. (Connolly)

In stark contrast with this stands the surge of anti-smoking legislation in the American Congress, partly reflecting the progress of the public health lobby and a weakening of the tobacco lobby's influence. Non-smoking has become the accepted norm in the US where there is considerable emphasis on the rights of non-smokers. Nevertheless the response of the tobacco interests – to target sales at women, minorities and poor people – tempers optimism.

It may seem obvious that the enemies of public health do not announce themselves and offer their corporate plans for open debate. There are two reasons why we need periodically to remind ourselves that some people and some firms make many people chronically ill and kill large numbers. First, when sponsorship is regarded simply as 'additional' or 'alternative' funding, it leads to dangerous naïvety, for instance, about the tobacco firms' motives for sponsoring the arts and sports; they receive praise as though they were public benefactors. They do not spend the firm's money for nothing. WHO's Expert Committee on Smoking Control concluded that tobacco was 'responsible for more than one million premature deaths each year' worldwide.

The second reason for recalling that accidents and illnesses are sometimes *manufactured* is the failure of many people who ought to know better, such as NHS staff, to make it impossible for governments to permit tobacco promotion and other public health obscenities. Their training omits anything to do with the politics of health. For example, medical and nursing students are typically given no idea of the nineteenth-century battles that had to be fought to separate sewage from drinking water, to end child labour in factories and to teach adults about birth control. Medical and nursing textbooks and lectures generally present students with a dull and misleading picture of progress in public health.

Disinformation

Public health partly depends on the public being kept aware of health hazards and what can be done about them. The mass media are obviously of critical importance but some British national newspapers function as disinformation battalions. This topic is discussed in Chapter 11, but a typical example of the scale of the problem is given here. *The Sun* excelled itself during the NHS cash crisis of 1987-88. An editorial (9 November 1987) announced that the NHS budget was a 'massive £20 million'. Eight days later page one said the total budget was 'almost £12 BILLION' while its editorial on the same day helpfully asked 'what on earth is the point of chucking another £100 million into the Health Service? . . . Alongside a £22 billion budget, it is a puddle compared with the Pacific'.

A special kind of enemy

These cases of damage to people's health by powerful producers are only the tip of a large iceberg – that network of Right-oriented policy think-tanks from both sides of the Atlantic and around the globe that supply enemies of health and safety with a common cause and a protective philosophy. Many of these think-tanks are as transnational in their operations as the corporate giants that finance them. Health has long been a prime target of these political *mafiosi*, as a number of attacks on the NHS from British groups has shown. The Adam Smith Institute's *Health Policy* is a typical example relevant to the latest Conservative NHS management destabilisation. Earlier and more comprehensively, the best-known organisation, the Washington-based Heritage Foundation, once described as the 'cutting edge of conservatism's renaissance in the United States', devoted a report to an attack on WHO. It defended the principles of private enterprise against Third World pressures on the rich countries for health aid commensurate with needs.

From 1974, when a UN General Assembly resolution called for a new international economic order to redress North-South economic inequality, WHO had faced hostility from an American business lobby at the UN – the International Chamber of Commerce – which had enjoyed consultative status since the world body was founded.

The Heritage Foundation was a main inspirer in the mid-1980s of attacks on WHO as part of the United Nations system, attacks that threatened its very existence. Multinational companies clearly felt WHO was cramping their style.

> . . . In spite of all this WHO at last managed to put out a particularly clear and strong message on smoking . . . Passive, enforced or involuntary smoking violates the right to health of non-smokers who must be protected against this noxious form of environmental pollution. (Anon. p. 1)

The London associate of the Heritage Foundation, the Adam Smith Institute, declared:

> Only the poor need the welfare state. If it can be shown that it has not helped them in the best way the present welfare state has lost its raison d'être.

The Heritage Foundation was started in 1973 and by 1988 its income had been lifted to £11 million a year by donations from companies. Its links with the Reagan team, in whose initial election programme it had a large hand, were extensive, no fewer than fifty-one of its former employees having had jobs at one time or another in Reagan administrations. Indeed, Right-wing policy groups blossomed under Reagan's presidency. *Labour Research* found 'an intricate network of personalities' involved with British groups:

> UK people with Heritage connections include Dr Stuart Butler (ASI) who is now director of domestic policy studies at the Heritage Foundation in the US. He co-edited the foundation's *Privatisation: a*

strategy for taming the federal budget, which outlined a strategy for turning eight government programmes over to the private sector.

In 1987 the *New Statesman* magazine revealed that the foundation was funding several organisations, including the London-based, pro-NATO, anti-CND Institute for European Defence and Strategic Studies. This Institute received £100,000 from the US group in 1985, and according to the US journal *Nation* £120,000 the next year. The Adam Smith Institute puts forward in Britain the policies of privatisation and cuts in government spending advocated by the Heritage Foundation.

In the US Accuracy in Media, another pressure group, has been dedicated to monitoring press and TV since 1969 to ensure that the Right's briefings are well used. Two self-appointed watchdogs of the British media, the Freedom Association and the Media Monitoring Unit have emulated the methods of Accuracy in Media to assist the Tory campaign, against TV in particular, over alleged Left bias. The chair of the Freedom Association, Norris McWhirter, told a meeting that after trade unions 'one of the greatest threats to freedom of thought and individual opinion is politically biased television beamed into 99.1 per cent of homes'.

Other obstacles

The battlefield analogy for the realities of much public health can take us too far if we begin to think that all the difficulties are essentially political in nature. Apart from what are clearly scientific or technical problems, such as the difficulties in developing an effective and safe vaccine against AIDS, there are other problems, that can be discussed in terms of factors that impede social change in healthier directions and policies that inadvertently cause health-damaging social change.

Bureaucratic inertia

The British TV satire of the 1980s, *Yes Minister*, became popular because it featured manipulation and trickery by senior civil servants and egocentric politicians. It showed that when such a bureaucratic elite exerts its considerable power, especially to resist change, the activities are political in nature but far from democratic, however much the Sir Humphreys pretend to be acting in the public interest.

In attempts to achieve what WHO calls healthy public policy (intersectoral policy, collaboration among sectors to promote health), a rather specialised field of management and sociological studies – the study of policy-making and implementation among organisations – becomes highly relevant. A review of inter-organisational research published by the WHO European region summarises the consensus of three studies about conditions conducive to the co-operation of large organisations in the following points:

- the fewer the participants the higher the chances they will co-operate
- the less co-operation required among ministries and agencies the better the relationships
- the less change that is involved the greater the likelihood of consensus and decision-making
- the greater political support and shared goals among policy sectors the more likely it is that they will co-operate and make joint decisions
- the fewer programme elements or programmes that have to be shared with other ministries the greater the probability that policy sectors will co-operate.
- the fewer resources needed from other ministries the greater the likelihood of co-operation
- the greater the gains (political and administrative) for all participating units, ministries and sectors the better the chances of co-operation. (Altenstetter)

Inadequate information

The development of health-promoting policy that is acceptable from other perspectives, such as its implications for finite resources, is often complex even at this conceptual level and without any consideration of how easy or difficult it would be to implement. This 'real life' factor must not be confused with problems that arise because earlier political decisions have obstructed the necessary research and development work. For example, better energy policy is currently very difficult to develop in Britain because research and development into renewable and non-polluting forms of energy production have been preached about rather than financed. Nevertheless the preachers always pretend to know all there is to know about the subject. In an extreme case, the Atomic Energy Authority at Harwell so distorted the cost of wave power that the Department of Energy withdrew £3 million from a key development project; the distortions were not admitted for eight years (Brown). Fortunately work done in several other countries provides a solid basis for ecologically-informed challenges to be mounted.

Intellectual blocks

Nowadays the concept of numeracy as well as literacy is widely understood; however, a basic understanding of ecological systems is also essential if policy-makers and electorates are to develop policies that make sense in terms of sustainable patterns of living. Although the Greening of electorates, policy-makers and politicians is now proceeding much more rapidly than ten to fifteen years ago, it is still much too slow in relation to the needs. Too many critical decisions are still being determined by the eco-blind – and in the land of the eco-blind, the money-greedy polluter is king.

Inadvertent damage to public health

An underlying aim of the EEC's Common Agricultural Policy was to safeguard employment in rural areas – clearly an acceptable aim in principle from a health viewpoint. However, with the benefit of subsequent nutritional research, it is also clear that this policy leaves a lot to be desired. It is a good example of a policy that is health-damaging on a significant scale but has innocent origins – at least in this respect. Knowledge accumulates that should render policies obsolete. This is common in health policy, for instance, with the slow establishment of the toxic effects of lead in petrol, the long-term effects of asbestos and so on. It is when the evidence mounts that people defending the *status quo* and their jobs and other economic interests generate an intensely political struggle. Tobacco presents a clear illustration.

Battles about health in a wider context

The problems of winning battles for people's health need to be understood in relation to how comparable social conflicts are handled. While some Britons are proud of their 'mother of parliaments', it is an open secret that much of the citizenry finds itself none too impressed with either the performances or the products. Think only of the quality of decision-making in ecological, economic, industrial, educational, transport or housing policy. It matters little where one starts, with the unelected Lords or the disproportional, whip-following Commons; both are trapped in rituals that mainly ratify decisions taken elsewhere – taken in Downing Street, in the Treasury, in Brussels and so on. Despite all the shouting and waving of order papers, despite all the trooping in and out of the division lobbies, despite all the petty, point-scoring, overgrown-schoolboy speeches and shouting in debates and at ritualised question times, significant change comes only here and there at best and more often from quiet all-party and collaborative work in committees rather than from the hours of sterile confrontation. Mrs Thatcher's governments in particular have shown that most of the power does not lie in the daily antics of the 'mother of parliaments'.

Compared with the possibilities of backbenchers actually changing things by investigations, discussions and negotiations as, for example, in the US Congress or Senate, the Nordic or Netherlands' parliaments, the Westminster scene tends to please only the Establishment and tourists. Indeed, parliamentary dysfunction was a principal reason for the setting up of Charter 88, which is discussed further in Chapter 11.

To turn from what are supposed to be the 'assemblies for peaceful conflict resolution' to some of the key decision-makers themselves. One reason why some ministers pursue policies that damage vulnerable people's health and well-being is their lack of relevant social experience. People like GPs, community nurses, social workers, home helps, teachers and clergy who frequently do home visits or have other regular contacts with the disadvantaged possess social knowledge that is rare not only in the Cabinet but in much wider circles of the Establishment. This may be one reason why some ministers, and Mrs Thatcher in particular, saw these pastoral roles as so threatening. Only on very rare occasions do ministers acknowledge their lack of social experience. An outstanding example was Peter Walker's confession after he had visited a multi-occupied house in Lambeth some years ago. To his eternal credit, he candidly admitted he did not know anyone was having to live in such conditions. His education, like that of many parliamentarians and senior civil servants, had scarcely been structured to foster even a glimmer of understanding of life at the bottom.

To end this discussion of politics and public health, a single but basic example sums up the impossibility of healthy public policy without a healthy body politic. In years to come the symbol of the feebleness of public health in the 1980s may come to be seen to be a closed public toilet. Whereas the Victorians went to all the trouble and expense of building those lavatorian monuments, the central and local politicians of the 1980s have so often failed to keep them open. The basic responsibility probably lies with ministers who relentlessly cut local powers and funds in the name of financial control, thereby increasing their own powers. Public toilets may not be *essential* for health reasons in the narrow sense of preventing gastrointestinal diseases. However, they cut risks and simple human well-being requires that conveniences – the word itself makes the point – be maintained and kept open.

In this British situation of creaking political machinery for the resolution of social conflicts and the development of ecologically prudent policies, it is not surprising that the most value-laden and political of the branches of health care – public health – should be going through a bad phase.

REFERENCES

C. Altenstetter, 'The Political, Economic and Institutional Prerequisites of Legislation and Planning in Support of Health Promotion', in T. Abelin, Z. Brzezinski and V. Carstairs (eds.), *Measurement in Health Promotion and Protection* (Copenhagen, WHO Regional Office for Europe, 1987).

Anon., 'WHO Refuses to Go Up in Smoke', *THS Health Summary*, May 1986.

P. Brown, 'Wave Power Undercuts Nuclear Cost', *The Guardian*, 1 June 1990.

Adam Smith Institute, *Health Policy* (London, Adam Smith Institute, 1984).

S. Chapman, *Cigarette Advertising and Smoking: A Review of the Evidence* (London, BMA, 1985).

G. Connolly, *Tobacco Politics and US Trade Policy* (Washington, 1987). Unpublished paper.

Labour Research Department, 'The Long Claws of the American Right', *Labour Research*, 77 (1988).

R. Nader, *Unsafe at Any Speed* (New York, 1965; London, 1973).

Office on Smoking and Health, *Smoking, Tobacco and Health: A Fact Book* (Washington, Dept. of Health and Human Services, 1987).

P. Taylor, *Smoke Ring: The Politics of Tobacco* (London, 1984).

J. Wilkinson, *Tobacco; The Facts Behind the Smokescreen* (Harmondsworth, 1986).

WHO Expert Committee on Smoking Control, *Controlling the Smoking Epidemic* (Geneva, WHO, 1983).

CHAPTER 8

Gender politics in the new public health

Hilary Rose

> *While some aspects of the health-influencing environment are*
> *very similar if not identical for men and women, for people of*
> *different ethnic groups and for people of different socio-*
> *economic groups, many other health-relevant aspects of the*
> *human environment vary strikingly with gender, race and class.*
> *This chapter focuses on gender issues, from cars to attacks on*
> *the Welfare State by the New Right, and how looking at*
> *poverty for households glosses over inequitable divisions*
> *within the household.*

Politics and health

> *Medicine is a social science, and politics are nothing else than*
> *medicine on a larger scale. (Rudolf Virchow)*

While in many ways men's and women's needs for a health-promoting
environment are the same, so that it makes sense to speak of general human
needs, it is also true that gender structures our lives, not least in terms of
differential patterns of morbidity and mortality. In consequence any discussion of the new public health has to include the specific needs of women.
The politics of sex, like those of 'race' and class, are integral to the politics of
health. Death by violence shows up in the statistics as caused by young
working class men, and in the US of young black working class men, but
violence by men against women, sexual harassment and rape, are also
matters of everyday reality which only begin to be reflected in the official
statistics in response to clear feminist political pressure. Without political
struggle which insists that a broken arm, a black eye or forced intercourse

are not ignorable natural events but reflect unequal relations between the genders, certain health problems would remain invisible and unaddressed.

Nor for that matter do black and Asian people merely live in poorer housing than white people and have worse paid jobs, they are also exposed to the violent racism of a recrudescent fascism. Thus in addition to the fires caused through the paraffin heaters and faulty wiring of poverty, semi-organised thugs put lighted brands through letter boxes and cause the deaths of entire households. Again only strong anti-racist pressure insists that these are not accidents to be passed over, but the unhealthy product of racialised social relations. More quietly, old people, particularly old women, die of so called fuel poverty, actually a blend of deficient British architecture and heating systems and too little cash. It seems scarcely surprising that women are more than twice as likely as men to be diagnosed as depressed, and working class and especially black people are several times more likely to be diagnosed as schizophrenic than middle class whites. It is not easy to be either sane or healthy in a racist and sexist society.

Whether we consider the health implications of poverty, unemployment, gender, transport, food policy, violence, energy or the contribution of the unpaid health watchdogs within the home, gender and 'race' politics are present and cannot be either subsumed under class or ignored. When the poverty or transport studies use access to a car as an indicator of a family's or household's wealth status, they reflect the global status of the unit of measurement, but fail to bring out that while 'he' takes the car to work, 'she' walks or queues, with 'their' children, for the bus. While ecologists might advocate the merits of the bus as a more environmentally-friendly solution, she, standing in the rain, might well be attracted by the claims of an ungreen liberal feminism which supports her claims for a car. An essay which tries to address the gender dimension of the politics of health has a choice. It is possible either to create an empirical litany of deprivation, which implicitly casts women as victims – or to begin the task of generating a political analysis of health and welfare which examines the balance of political forces and explores whether and how feminists and their allies might move towards health as politics. This essay chooses the latter approach.

Prospects for health

The current situation, despite the many and obvious dangers, is not without real chances for health. The hope comes from both outside and inside the old capitalist societies, not least our own. Outside, the 'evil empire' is dissolving, and it is increasingly difficult politically to organise huge military structures and continuously court the possibility of global war.* Peace becomes more a concrete possibility and less a continued statistical accident; in consequence it is important to consider – to use today's market language – what should be done with the peace dividend (Editorial). Real resources become available and must be used for producing health and well-being, not squandered in, for example, tax handouts to the rich.

This is not to say that anyone can be sure whether the quickly stirred cocktail of a longing for freedom, nationalism, and an infatuation with the market will produce health and well-being for Eastern Europe, but at least the nightmare of the unthinkable recedes. While it seems easier to argue as a poet than as a social scientist that we have become freer from collective bomb psychosis, the new situation offers a chance that even a year ago seemed impossible. But anti-militarists and feminists have to remember that while it made sense to chant at the Greenham wire 'take the toys from the boys', and to make the connections between masculinity and militarism, a healthy public policy requires that viable and socially useful jobs are developed for the military and the bombmakers as necessarily as for the coca farmers of Latin America or the tobacco workers of the world. The dividend of peace must be made to support health for all.

The second positive chance which comes from both outside and inside is in the threat of global warming. Nature, so long exploited and dominated above all by the countries of the North, now replies. Whilst scientists continue to debate the certainty of the threat, politicians vie in their claims to be Green, industry sells us 'Green' products, and people, and particularly young people, seem to be moving to the defence of nature.

This weakening of the risk of global war and the strengthening of the necessity to live pacifically with nature constitutes a double chance to create a healthy society. While I do not claim that women are naturally near to nature and naturally non-violent, it is true that most feminists claim that feminist values are less violent, more pacific towards people and nature than those of masculinism. Feminism's ally, the Green movement, speaks of an ecological science and politics which take care of rather than exploit and dominate the environment. If the science which has underpinned the technologies of violence between people, and between people and nature, is to be reformed so as to serve the ends of health, the values and visions of these new social movements will be a crucial ingredient.

At the same time, inside the rather small country of Britain, with its limping economy, weakened democratic forms and highly authoritarian government, there is also a ferment of small community-based groups

---

*When this was written I did not think that the US, having successfully blockaded Nicaragua – which had a good deal going for it in health policy terms – would spearhead a UN force against Iraq without using the blockade strategy to the hilt.

dealing with common problems, as was noted in Chapter 1. Typically focused on single issues, they may be concerned with a shared health condition, a polluting factory or a dangerous road; they may not even think of themselves as working on health-related issues. On the whole rather pragmatic, they may work close to, outside or against the official health system (Hatch and Kickbusch). For that matter such self-help groups move rather swiftly between these three approaches, the consensual, the conflictual and the alternative. While some remain at the level of purely self-help, enabling members of a small local group to cope, others defend or seek to extend the existing health care provisions, and yet others seek to move towards a more supportive healthy society.

The necessity of confronting the AIDS epidemic has seen the gay movement involved with all three forms of activity. First it had to develop fast and effective health education among the gay community – in Britain well before there was official cognisance of the significance of AIDS. Simultaneously, it had to contest a virulent homophobia, orchestrated by sections of the media against the 'gay plague' and finally, with the help of a number of committed professionals, work to protect the health and citizenship rights of people with HIV/AIDS. In 1990 the international gay movement, faced with visa restrictions on sero-positive people within and without the US, organised a massive international boycott of the San Francisco AIDS research conference. This boycott, of a meeting held in a city at the forefront of AIDS work, was intended to show that the struggle for the human rights of people with AIDS is integral with and not separable from the struggle for equal access to good quality health care, research and all the rest.

The feminist movement has a comparable relationship with the women's health movement. Thus while the women's health movement consists of a multiplicity of groups offering well women centres and mutual support in coping with specific health issues, and tackling women's homelessness, at intervals, usually because of a fresh challenge by the so-called pro-life groups, it comes together with all of feminism to defend women's health and right to abortion. That fundamental and infectious question of feminism – 'Whose body is it anyway?' inspires women to reclaim control over their own bodies against masculine and medical dominance. This question has touched some very general nerve of body justice for the great majority of the population, as numerous opinion surveys show support for this basic right.

Women and welfare

A new public health which seeks in a systematic way to address the social, the political and the economic as well as the natural environments through which women's health and illness are produced, has to begin with a working analysis, from the perspective of women, of the impact of the New Right on the public provision of health and welfare services. The changes have had particular significance in women's lives. The last decade has witnessed nothing less than a counter-revolution by the New Right against the old Welfare State. This counter-revolution was intended to dismantle the public provision of welfare and some health services, and in depressingly large measure has succeeded. Public services, above all housing, that foundation for everyday healthy living, have been replaced with what has been described euphemistically as the 'new welfare mix'. This new mix speaks of services provided through the market to those who can afford them, with, but this is left unsaid, second class public services for those who cannot. Some services have been allocated to community care as part of a general social project of restoring the 'family' or 'Victorian' values.

As many vulnerable people have outlived their families, have no family or have lost touch with them, community care exists more at the level of rhetoric than in actuality (Finch and Groves). And where it does exist, community care, particularly at the hard end of coping with daily double incontinence, rather than the soft end of sweeping away snow for an elderly neighbour, is mainly carried out by women. Even where the 'new man' shows signs of emerging, his care work is mainly reported with young children, rather than with old or profoundly challenged people. It is not by chance that the beautiful young man in the poster is pictured with a naked newborn baby, not with an old and dying person. The policy of 'community care' at its most visible and most scandalous has been in relation to the mentally ill, who have been evicted from residential care and made homeless along with others the State has abandoned, literally living and dying on the streets. Even there the habit of caring clings on; workers with homeless people consistently report that homeless women, out of their non-existent resources, still try to take care of homeless men.

The point of discussing this counter-revolution is not simply to express anger at the abandonment of people who need care. Rather, it is to grasp what this means for the lives of women in the 1990s and thus its implication for the formation of a new woman-friendly public health. In this new public health is the possibility of a new 'welfare society', which is neither based on the premise of systematically unequal relations between men and women nor racist, but moves beyond both the statism of the old Welfare State and also the crudities and cruelties of Thatcherism and the New Right. It is neither possible to go back to the old Welfare State, nor to continue as at present. We need to insist that a new social project, offering a new vision of a society which people can see is both good and gettable, is urgently required.

In thinking about a future society it is important to recognise that women's well-being has been tied up in a very particular way with the history of the old Welfare State, whether we recollect the slow haul through the nineteenth and early twentieth century in the old industrial countries or begin with the long economic boom extending from post-war reconstruction up to the economic crisis of the mid 1970s. In Britain these post-war years represented the full maturity of the Welfare State, with the NHS its much vaunted jewel in the crown. Even while we defend the NHS as an efficient method of providing curative services, we also rightly criticise it both as coercive, with far too much power given to the male-dominated medical profession, and as failing to promote health. Less familiar may be the feminist critique of both the old Welfare State and the NHS as constraining women, so that the real benefits women received from its provisions have always had to be set against the dependency on men they enforced.

Looking back at the original Beveridge/Keynes model, it is now easy to see that it offered the Labour movement full employment – in actuality for men and for single, but not married, women – and the public provision of social services, with a societal commitment to the provision of welfare beneath which no citizen was to be permitted to fall. In return the Labour movement was to provide social peace in which a modified capitalism could continue with the fundamental and unchanged task of capital accumulation. In this model men were to be the husbands/fathers and breadwinners through their place in the labour market, and women were to be the wives/mothers, the carers and dependents of men in the home. He was to become the first class citizen in the new society, she the second class citizen whose benefits from the cradle to the grave depended on a male other. This historic post-war settlement, supported with varying degrees of enthusiasm by the main political parties together with the trade union movement, constituted a powerful political consensus – above all among men. Its ideological grip was eventually weakened during the last Labour government by Callaghan's and Healey's retreat from Keynesian economic policies as a means of managing the economic crisis of the 1970s, and decisively broken by the advent of the Thatcher government in 1979. Thatcherism saw the Welfare State as no longer the handmaid of capital accumulation but its impediment.

But the old Welfare State had also contained the seeds of its own change, for the provision of services which supported women's unpaid work as carers at the same time provided new employment opportunities for married women. Where the Welfare State had begun as a story in which women were cast as the dependents of men, as the story developed, women increased their independence. It can be read as the shift from private patriarchy, in which women depended on a particular man, whether a father or a husband, to a public patriarchy in which women depended on a masculinist state (Hernes). The attack on welfare over the past decade has therefore affected women twice over; first they lost in terms of the reduced services available to support their work as the primary carers and health promoters within the family, and secondly they lost as Welfare State employees. Either the jobs within health and welfare are lost altogether, or they are relocated in the market sector through privatisation, with, in all too many cases, rather worse conditions of employment. It is not by chance that in the opinion polls women are more supportive than men of public welfare provision, for its existence affects women's lives very much more directly.

The counter-revolution by the New Right has sought to turn the clock back from the relative freedom of the public patriarchy to the intimate oppression of the private patriarchy, or, in the inimitable language of the New Right, through the restoration of 'Victorian values'. These values were of course symbolised for women by a capital city in which the main chances of employment for working class women were as servants or as prostitutes, and where for middle class women any form of personal development, above all education, was resisted as a mental and gynaecological health hazard. Thus the British New Right has fused two uneasy strands of conservative thought, the traditionalist and the market-liberal, which together add up to bad news for women.

It would be wrong to underestimate the criticism of the Welfare State by those who were supposed to be its beneficiaries and the extent to which the anti-Welfare State politics of the New Right initially won popular support, not least amongst the skilled working class. However, it is now abundantly clear what price is being paid, and by whom, for its near destruction. Evidence concerning the extent of the damage should ideally encompass all those measures of command over the resources for daily living, from access to clean water, fresh air, decent housing, safe streets, employment with good working conditions, to access to good quality health and welfare services. In actual fact when Right wing politics crush feelings of social solidarity, the complexity of demands diminishes and the possibility of connected healthy public policies recedes; the core of the debate retreats to the distribution of income and wealth, death and illness – above all to the incidence of poverty, as the simplest and crudest indicator of access to health and well-being in any given society.

Women and poverty

Early in 1990, when directors of leading banks and industrial firms were seen to be allocating themselves pay rises of some 30 per cent and more, generating annual salaries of £300,000 to £500,000, there was an immediate and outraged contrast drawn with the desperate world of cardboard city. While it is true that opinion polls during the 1980s have reflected more social concern than the government or the media showed, the latter – though not the former – seem to be relinquishing their support for unbounded greed and consumerism. But not only has the government declared war on the poor, it has also suppressed the evidence of their existence. While this erasure is important to the well-being of all low-income people, it is particularly important to women because they are massively over-represented among the poor.

Two recent studies carried out by the Institute of Fiscal Studies on behalf of the Commons Social Services Committee show that in 1988 an estimated one in five British people lived in or on the margins of poverty (Johnson and Webb). This suggested that the new income support system, implemented in 1988, despite the government's language of efficiency and 'targeting' which accompanied its introduction, is failing to find and help low-income people. It estimates that 0.8 million fewer people received safety net help in 1988 than in the last year of the old system. What we are experiencing is not only policies cruelly indifferent to the health and well-being of poor and vulnerable people, but a policy process where truth is a mere incidental casualty. Contrary to the view of Mrs Thatcher's former most senior civil servant, Sir Robert Armstrong, we cannot be economical with the truth, as honest social statistics are a crucial aid to a healthy and democratic society.

But while feminists share the legitimate concern about the blunting of the tools for the management of a healthy and democratic society, they also challenge both the way in which poverty statistics are compiled and the traditions of poverty research that still mask the extent of poverty within families which, when viewed as units, are above the poverty line. While taxation in the form of income tax moves partially towards accepting the individual adult as the unit of assessment, poverty research still aggregates the household/family – it, not individuals within it, constitutes the unit of assessment.

Even though the history of the gender division of welfare within the home, from the allocation of the best food to that of leisure – whether in the form of a pint of beer in the pub or a workout at the sports centre – is full of examples showing that men secure an unequal share, the mainstream (male stream?) poverty literature of both government and opposition assume that behind the family door all is equity. Feminist research of the past fifteen years indicates that such an assumption is as absurd as to assume that there was equity between the classes within the old Welfare State. But then, as G.D.H. Cole argued many years ago, the problem is not one of poverty but of powerlessness – Cole's point being not a denial of the reality of poverty but a reminder of its political causes and the political reasons for its persistence.

From both personal and historical experience we know that power is not usually given by the powerful to the powerless, but has to be taken, usually in the face of fierce resistance. Today's talk of empowerment, not least in health circles, sometimes moves close to sounding like fashionable head-games rather than the struggle for power through which the real and material resources which guarantee a better chance of health may be won. Women need equality of access to the labour market, and a radically reformed labour market where better conditions such as generally shorter hours and safe working conditions support family life. Bottom-line benefits, such as child benefit and state pensions, are crucial to women's empowerment. With adequate child benefit women have increased control over the production of health and welfare for their children; with adequate pensions women in old age have a measure of independence from children and the helping professions. For despite the hype of the new private pensions located in the stylish post-feminist discourse of the finance industry, there can be few sanguine hopes about the pensions future of women. For the current generation of women in paid work, the erosion of state pensions and the expansion of private sector pensions are predicated on a situation in which their employment involves regular full-time jobs unbroken by child rearing, which will enable them to build up occupational or private pensions in their own right.

Nor has the situation of the majority of women – to say nothing of the many poorer women – been much helped by the consumerist politics of the 1980s. Designer healthism has little to say to, or for, most women. The potentially universalist language of health for all, with its friendly talk of making the healthy choice the easy choice, inviting public policy makers to facilitate a mass healthy life style, has been almost appropriated by an individualist view of lifestyle. For most women, coping with the double demands of family and employment is a daily precarious balancing act. Women's lives are carried out in that space between the private and the public, endlessly enabling, endlessly making connections, so that their coping or not coping seems to become the central signal as to whether they, and those who depend on them, are making out. Such a coping, piecemeal, everyday life does not of itself form the basis of a powerful and coherent social movement which can feed in any straightforward way into the demands for a more supportive, healthier society. It cannot reproduce the clarity of the old Labour movement which so successfully pressed for the 1945 Welfare State; the pressures will be experienced as complex and diffuse, and the new structures of public health will need to reflect that complexity.

Thus a reinvented public health cannot just add women and stir. There is no possibility of tacking women's demands, preferably presented as a tidy coherent list, onto some 'masterplan' for a new public health agenda which presides over and above all the political arenas. Gender politics both crudely and subtly penetrate every area of public policy and everyday living. In consequence while feminists can raise issues from poverty to the environment and show that these affect women in particular ways, it is only when men as well as women understand that the social production of health and illness is a profoundly gendered process that a new public health moves beyond, rather than reproduces, the old politics and the old medicine. Moving this recognition of gender politics into the 'art and the science of public health' is going to be an exciting task, in itself producing healthier and more equitable social relations between the people who work to reinvent it.

REFERENCES

E. Ackernecht, *Rudolf Virchow* (New York, 1981). The nineteenth century public health reformer Virchow argued that it was important to study the cells, the organism and its total environment.

Editorial, *Social Policy*, Spring/Summer 1990.

J. Finch and D. Groves (eds.), *A Labour of Love* (London, 1986).

S. Hatch and I. Kickbusch (eds.), *Self Help and Health in Europe* (Copenhagen, WHO Regional Office for Europe, 1983).

H. Hernes, 'Women and the Welfare State: The Transition from Private to Public Dependence', in H. Holter (ed.), *Patriarchy in a Welfare Society* (Oslo, 1984).

Paul Johnson and Steven Webb, *Households and Families below Average Income: A Regional Analysis* (London, 1990).

Paul Johnson and Steven Webb, *The Income Support System and the Distribution of Income in 1987* (London, 1990).

CHAPTER 9

Economics and hostile environments

Victor Anderson and Peter Draper

*In understanding economic factors in today's hostile
environments, the thesis is that conventional economics
provides misleading assessments of social costs (such as those
of pollution and damaging unemployment), of economic
progress or growth, and of work – socially useful activity,
including that of 'housewives', unemployed people and
voluntary organisations.*

*Avoidable health hazards are scrutinised under the economist's
categories of production, distribution and consumption. Myths
about the economy are then dissected: what is economic or
uneconomic with more comprehensive accounting; the
deceptive assumptions in the assessments of Gross National/
Domestic Product; some of the ways in which economics is far
from neutral.*

*Finally, a brief review of health economics moves on to
assessing projects for a Green or 'new' economics, outside the
monetarist or Keynesian mainstreams and Marxist or other
political economy.*

The economy as a danger to health

In what ways do our patterns of consumption avoidably damage our
health? Considering first the diseases or risks that are primarily related to
the nature of consumption, some clear examples are the tobacco diseases,
road accidents due to the consumption of alcohol or other drugs, damage of
our health through the use of leaded petrol, and the increased risk of skin
cancer from the use of aerosol sprays with chlorofluorocarbons which
damage the ozone layer.

What we consume can also affect our health adversely through the level of consumption. Advertising that seduces or otherwise pressures us to consume more than is good for us, whether it is food or alcohol, is one illustration. Equally, advertising that in effect stamps obsolete on household goods or clothes contributes to domestic pressures to keep up with the Joneses. This surreptitiously erodes well-being. Another kind of hazard, relentlessly accumulating damage, comes from unhealthy patterns of eating among schoolchildren, particularly since the 1980 Education Act abolished nutritional standards for school meals: there are problems of insufficient intake, for instance of Vitamin C, or excess intake, such as of sugar and animal fats, which arise for example from a daily lunch consisting mainly of items such as icecream, crisps, chips and doughnuts.

Damage to health occuring in production, can also be looked at in terms of the nature or level of the activity. Any abandonment or circumventing of health and safety procedures to save time or money, as happens for instance in some road haulage firms so that rest periods are not taken (BBC), shows how the rate of work or level of production can be a health hazard. Health and safety factors at work fall into two broad categories: direct factors such as exposure to toxic chemicals, radiation or unsafe machinery and indirect ones such as the tendency to produce de-skilling, unemployment and two classes of worker: one skilled, secure and well-paid and the other de-skilled or unskilled, badly paid and insecure. In the second category, as is clear from contrasts with other European countries, we are dealing with an avoidably hostile socio-economic environment that has adverse consequences for health.

The realisation that human socio-economic environments can be health-damaging seems to come slowly – if at all – to people who have no experience or understanding of poverty. And it is crucial to understanding public health in Britain to be aware that this includes many people in high places, many senior civil servants as well as ministers, judges and magistrates, for instance. Yet today's poverty is the central issue in considering how the distribution of income and wealth affect health. Before we look at four of the major studies of inequalities and health in rich countries that followed the publication of the Black Report (1980), it is relevant to note that the health improvements achieved in some poor countries through socio-economic measures have been striking. Werner commented forcefully but reasonably:

As has been demonstrated in China, Cuba, Nicaragua, Kerala State in India, and elsewhere, the health of a nation's people has more to do with fair distribution of resources than with total wealth. Fair distribution, in turn, depends upon egalitarian government. What it comes down to is that the health of the poor in the world today is abysmal because too many governments are in the hands of powerful, elite groups, or military juntas, that do not fairly represent their people. Clearly, what is needed is radical change, of governments and social structures. Those who rule the world today will not bring about the changes that are needed for the wellbeing of the people. They have too much self-interest in maintaining the status quo. The changes can only come about through organised action of the people themselves. In most countries today, primary health care implies a very fundamental, social evolution – if not revolution.

In rich countries evidence built up during the 1980s about the adverse effects of socio-economic disadvantage on people's health. For example, Whitehead, who updated the analyses of the Black Report, concludes:

The evidence . . . confirms that serious social inequalities in health have persisted . . . Whether social position is measured by occupational class, or by assets such as house and car-ownership, or by employment status . . . Those at the bottom of the social scale have much higher death rates than those at the top . . . at every stage of life from birth, through adulthood and well into old age . . . health inequalities between social groups are genuine and cannot be explained away as an artefact. (pp. 1-3)

But are these differences explained by the fact that some people move down the social scale *because* of their poor health? Whitehead reviews evidence for that view and concludes that it is not enough to explain the big differences in health between social groups. She points to recent in-depth studies that have

. . . increased understanding of how living and working conditions can impose severe restrictions on an individual's ability to choose a healthy life-style. They have provided fresh insight into the way behaviours are influenced by social conditions and argue for a policy which recognises the link between the two, in preference to policies which focus solely on the individual. (pp. 3-4)

In a review from the University of Helsinki of recent European work on the relationships of socio-economic position and death rates, Valkonen writes:

The greater part of socio-economic mortality differences is not caused by specific risk factors or inequalities in health care but by the general inequality of living conditions and related differences in life styles . . . The WHO document on *Targets for Health for All* comes to the same conclusion when it states: 'Most of the differences in health status are determined by living and working conditions'.

In another analysis of cross-sectional and longitudinal studies of income and mortality, Wilkinson comments 'there can be little doubt that substantial health benefits could be expected to accrue from a policy of income redistribution in Britain'. The BMA's Board of Science and Education examined socio-economic disadvantage and its impact on health and came to a similar conclusion:

In the short term, initiatives such as health education and screening campaigns are indicated and may improve health by intervening in the processes that cause disease. However, such measures do not affect the underlying problem of deprivation. In the interest of justice and public health, there should be a commitment to combat extreme social inequalities with the aim of eliminating deprivation.

Toward a health-promoting economy

From even these few illustrations of avoidable damage to people's health which occurs directly or as a side-effect of economic activity, the outline of a health-promoting or health-enhancing economy emerges clearly. The need is not that 'health should dictate all policy' but rather that the impact of any measure on people's health should be given some attention – as much as is given to the defence of the realm.

While it is easy to see some of the basic features of an economy that would promote health, some of the far-reaching changes would be far from easy to achieve politically. For instance, if health were to be given more priority, new patterns of development in Third World countries would have to be adopted by the transnational companies, the IMF, the World Bank and other international agencies. They would need to encourage the growing of food rather than cash crops such as tobacco. This is how a senior public health officer in Pakistan commented:

Tobacco growing is one of Pakistan's most important cash crops and an important source of government revenue . . . Approximately 120,000 acres of Pakistan's most fertile land is under tobacco cultivation. The cigarette industry is expanding. Cigarette consumption has been increasing at 8 per cent a year. Lung cancer is now the most common form of tumour found in men. (Taylor).

In passing, we should note that the spreading of tobacco addiction in the Third World and elsewhere is counted positively by orthodox economists because of the associated economic activity!

In contrast to the kill-joy image promoted by enemies of public health, health-enhancing economic policies would need to make the healthier choices easier choices. They would do so, for instance, by banning all advertisements for tobacco and alcohol. If someone produced a superb new alcoholic drink, publicans and restaurateurs would be only too glad to stock and recommend it. The message would get through all right. Interestingly, publicans are already doing quite a lot for the health and lives of their customers by making it easier to satisfy hunger with food rather than drink: an improvement on the position ten to fifteen years ago. Publicans who provide smoke-free areas are also helping. Making it normal to be able to have good coffee, unadulterated fruit juices and mineral waters at reasonable prices would be another breakthrough.

Besides implausible allegations that a health-enhancing economy would have doctors running everything – and kill-joy doctors at that – what other objections are commonly raised? Immediate resistance comes from people who simply do not see the connections that link, for instance, health with agriculture, fishing or transport. This seems to arise partly from lack of experience or imagination and partly from psychological patterns of thought that converge – however brilliantly – whereas lateral links are rarely seen. Astonishingly, and as we noted in the first chapter, Conservative ministers who have often denied any causal connection between extensive unemployment and drug-taking, between unemployment and other kinds of poverty we have today and ill-health, are given to crow about the NHS 'treating more patients than ever' as though the burden of accidents and illnesses borne by a population is unchanging and as though more activity in the repair shops was an infallible sign of public health success. In some ways the teaching of orthodox economics and accountancy and the seepage of such blinkered perspectives into everyday life encourage this kind of cerebral pigeon-holing or lateral blindness.

Other opponents of health-promoting economic policy say 'even if it might be a good idea, we couldn't afford it'. This has long been a stock objection to environmental measures that eventually came to be seen as basic, like keeping sewage out of the water supply and thick smoke or lead out of the air. As was demonstrated with smoke control in Britain, one of the key strategies for the public health and ecological lobbies is to get realistic costs for some of the externalities or side-effects – like the damage to buildings, the costs of treating the additional respiratory diseases – and above all for the money-obsessed, some cash assessments for the tremendous social losses, including the premature deaths.

Another objection comes from people who say 'perhaps we could afford the changes proposed, but who wants to live in a society with a big public health bureaucracy? We can't plan and control everything!'. Quite, but this is not what is proposed in having what are sometimes called health impact assessments of economic policy. This kind of opposition begins by making a bogey out of office staff in public services and by ignoring the many large private bureaucracies. Try telling a big insurance firm or a transnational that it does not need planning and other bureaucracies. In this context of cries of 'Bureaucracy!' it is salutary in passing to recall that if those objectors (the kinds of people who advocate commercial health insurance and medicine), were successful and abolished the NHS, simply to maintain the existing volume of clinical treatment would add about 20 per cent to the nation's health bill in order to support the kinds of insurance and hospital bureaucracies judged necessary in the US. And as in any well-run insurance firm, all the 'bad risks' – people in most need – would be excluded or offered insurance only at high premiums. As we shall see in the next section, what is in the narrow interests of the company, what is 'businesslike' or 'economic', is not necessarily in the public interest.

Myths about the economy

From brief case histories illustrating socio-economic harm to health and outlining principles through which health-enhancement policies could avoid the harm, we go on to examine the central objection that government and officialdom keep in stock to prevent such an expansion of public health horizons: that is, that it is 'uneconomic', beyond our means, so *ipso facto* ruled out.

This was the blunderbuss that, waved against the National Union of Miners, provoked the 1984-85 strike. Long before it was all over the dubiousness of the National Coal Board's argument that a substantial number of pit closures was economically mandatory had become widely apparent. The Board presented figures comparing wage costs plus operating costs with revenue from sales of coal and proving, it claimed, that many pits were 'loss-making'. But for whom? A loss for the NCB was quickly shown to be not necessarily one for the government.

The NCB, its employees and its suppliers all pay tax and national insurance contributions and closing pits would reduce government income. The consequent redundancies would increase government spending on unemployment benefit. Detailed calculations presented by Andrew Glyn in his *The Economic Case Against Pit Closures* showed that, considering the combined effect of the NCB's gains and the government's losses, not one pit was uneconomic. The accounting might also be taken some stages further: pit closures would tend to reduce coal production, thereby increasing the demand for oil, which would increase the price of oil, which would tend to increase the exchange rate of the pound, which would make it relatively cheaper for investors to buy assets overseas, which would be damaging to the balance of payments . . . and so on. Everything in the economy affects everything else, no element can be isolated. That must be taken into account before any conclusions should be reached about sacking people.

We must also take into account the ways in which the method of calculation of unemployment was altered in Britain to minimise the count, the practice of counting the proceeds from privatisation as 'negative expenditure' to make government spending look lower, and changes in the measures used for money supply.

The government is able through its command of the collection of statistics to see the whole picture, at least on a national scale. But what do the statistics measure? They add up the annual revenue of firms and nationalised industries and call the total Gross National Product. Production is valued at what people pay for it, so its total value must equal the revenue of firms and nationalised industries. If GNP goes up (after taking off the effects of price inflation), it is known as 'economic growth'. If the rate of growth is high, the economy is said to be 'successful'. If it is low, it is said to be 'stagnant'. High or low, if it is lower than the rate of most other countries, the country is said to be in 'relative decline'.

The various parts of the economy impose costs on other parts. Every time money is paid out for something the amount is added to the GNP. If a factory pollutes a river so that more people decide to buy bottled drinking water, production is said to have increased. If crime increases, causing more police to be employed, GNP goes up. If baby foods are promoted so that fewer infants are breastfed, that is also economic growth.

On the other hand, GNP ignores any creative activity that is not paid for. Output is valued at the prices paid. Since I do not pay myself for cooking a meal, it is said not to be 'productive'. But if I eat out and pay someone else for cooking it, then that meal counts toward the GNP. If I have some ailment that I treat myself with herbs from the garden, that does nothing for the GNP. But if I go to a consultant and pay, then what I pay gets counted. A large proportion of the work done by women in the home, including childcare, is unpaid and therefore plays no part in the GNP statistics.

Most production involves the use of resources, many of them limited in supply. The faster they can be sold, or used in production, the more is added to GNP. But the stock of resources available for future production is depleted. North Sea oil production, for example, was in the late 1980s directly contributing about 6 per cent to GNP. The faster oil is pumped out, the higher the GNP will go – in the short-term – but the lower it will tend to be in the future. No judgements can be made about the 'success' or 'failure' of an economy without some attempt to look at it long-term. That is only possible on the basis of information on the available reserves of the resources on which production depends. New economic indicators are needed that would give that information.

As well as reflecting resource depletion, 'growth' may reflect the rate at which goods are falling apart. Goods that depreciate and goods that break down create demand for replacement goods. The new goods count in the GNP; nothing gets subtracted for the loss of use of the previous set of goods. There should be some way of taking into account the average length of the useful life of goods, so that planned obsolescence or other reductions in this average life are seen as economic 'failure', not part of economic 'success' as now.

GNP ignores all the things that people value but do not buy. If, for example, I prefer to do one job rather than another that I might do at a higher salary, it is probably because I think that the loss in job satisfaction from changing to the higher-paid job would be greater than the financial gain. There is a sense in which I am prepared to 'pay for' the job I prefer doing. But because I am not actually buying anything, nothing is registered in the GNP statistics. If, nevertheless, I do change jobs, my income will increase, and therefore GNP will tend to rise, even though I am in a wider sense worse off. A high level of GNP may reflect the fact that a lot of people are doing jobs they would prefer not to be doing.

Similarly, people are frequently faced with a choice between having time off and using that time to earn more money. When they choose (non-spending) leisure they contribute to economic 'stagnation'. When they choose paid work they contribute to 'growth'. While it often makes sense for an individual to choose not to work overtime, or to choose part-time rather than full-time employment, a government that chose 'stagnation' rather than 'growth' would make itself very unpopular, but its choice might be just as rational.

In *Social Limits to Growth* Fred Hirsch drew attention to a further problem with economic growth by using the concept of 'positional goods'. These derive their value from the fact that other people do not have them – for example, my right to sit on a private beach is worth paying for because not everyone has the same right. Once everyone has it, it becomes worth nothing. Similarly, academic qualifications fall in their value to those who have them when more people get them. In the economy as a whole, if the output of these positional goods rises, their value must automatically fall, including the value of those already bought and paid for. It makes sense for the individual to pay for the benefits derived from positional goods. But it makes no sense for the government to add up the prices paid for such goods, count it in the GNP, and regard it as some sort of measure of the merits of its economic policies. The total sales of positional goods are more a measure of the degree of competitiveness in society.

For these and many other reasons, there has been increasing criticism in recent years of the concept of GNP (and the associated concept of GDP, to which all the criticisms given here also apply). Proposals have been put forward for replacing GNP, or supplementing it with alternative economic indicators. For example, the Labour Party statement on the environment, which became party policy at its 1986 conference, stated: 'Alongside indicators such as gross national product, we will introduce new economic indicators that take the environment and resource depletion into account'. The final World Conference of the United Nations Decade for Women, meeting in Nairobi in 1985, drew attention to the problem of unpaid and uncounted women's work in its document summing up the decade: 'The remunerated and, in particular, the unremunerated contributions of women to all aspects and sectors of development should be recognised, and appropriate efforts should be made to measure and reflect these contributions in national accounts and economic statistics and in the gross national product'. This document, 'Forward Looking Strategies', was agreed by the UN General Assembly on 6 November 1985. The Norwegian, French and other governments already use environmental indicators to supplement GNP. A policy judged to be a failure by the GNP indicator may become a success when considered in the light of an alternative indicator. In choosing to use GNP as a yardstick, governments and economists are making a whole series of implicit choices about what sorts of economic policies they prefer. They usually tend to deny this by referring to the 'neutral' and 'objective' nature of economics as a 'science'. The 'scientific' nature of economics has become one of the most influential myths of our time. To uncover the origins and implications of this myth, it is necessary to look into the history of economics and political economy.

Bias a constant in economics

First, a few statements of the myth itself. In his influential *An Essay on the Nature and Significance of Economic Science*, Lionel Robbins stated that economics is entirely neutral as between ends. This is reflected in the opening chapters of numerous textbooks, for example:

The determination of policies lies in the province of politics; it is the politician's function to decide policy matters. The economist's role in policy making is to act as an adviser, using specialist knowledge to provide policy makers with an analysis of the likely economic effects of the policy proposals . . . when economists pronounce on the desirability of any economic policy they have moved out of the field of economic analysis – they are making a value judgement. (G.F. Stanlake, *Introductory Economics*, Chapter 1)

The logic of setting up a division of labour in which economists are trained in a horror of value judgements is as follows: economics is a science, sciences exclude values, therefore economics excludes values, therefore when economists include values they are not acting as economists, but in some other capacity. Historically, this argument has been part of the attempt by practitioners of the 'social sciences' to set themselves up as proper scientists, imitating as far as possible the model of the natural sciences.

Eighteenth-century political economy (the most influential representative of which was Adam Smith) was closely associated with the Enlightenment and with the high value placed by the Enlightenment on reason and science. Political economy was, nevertheless, concerned with moral issues and values, and with the relationship between economic aspects of society and those aspects now distinguished as 'sociological' and 'political'. Most of the major contributors to political economy wrote on a very wide range of topics: Adam Smith preferred not to apply to his own work the increasing division of labour which he analysed so favourably elsewhere.

What completely changed the nature of economics – in fact, created economics in place of political economy – was the marginalist revolution of the 1870s. This established the neoclassical orthodoxy that still dominates mainstream economics today. On the basis of a small set of assumptions, the marginalists were able to draw out by mathematical and logical inference a large number of implications. They established to their own satisfaction the efficiency of 'perfect competition', free trade, the division of labour, the market economy, and so on.

Neoclassical economics developed to a large extent as a reaction against the economic analysis of Ricardo and Marx. Marxists continued to describe what they were doing as 'political economy', making explicit reference to political commitment in their work. Their opponents in what has become mainstream economics chose to describe their own work as non-political and scientific. For the neoclassical economists, 'scientific' meant both an absence of value judgements and the presence of a large quantity of mathematics. In both respects, they tried to emulate the natural sciences.

In the 1930s and 1940s, this process was taken a stage further. The most influential set of equations became Keynesian rather than neoclassical. The reception and application of Keynesian economics was greatly influenced by the neoclassical emphasis on mathematics. Keynes was very much in the old political economy tradition of someone who wrote about moral and political issues, and was concerned with philosophy and art, but his ideas came to be used as the basis for further mathematicisation of economics. Using Keynesian arguments and conclusions, the central features of the economy were set out in a series of equations: Y (national income) equals C (consumption) plus S (saving), etc. Gross National Product is essentially a Keynesian concept, which had to be calculated so that there were figures for Y to put in the equation.* More recently, the equations and the statistics to fit them have been put on computers, and forecasts made about what will happen. The quantity theory of money has been developed into a rival set of monetarist equations, with its own statistics and forecasts.

There have therefore been three main stages in the development of economics as a mathematically-based 'science': its initial association with the Enlightenment tradition in the eighteenth century, the marginalist revolution in the nineteenth century, and the Keynesian revolution of the twentieth century. However, the more quantitative it has become in its emphasis, the less consideration it has given to features of the economy that are difficult to measure and put into equations. Far from creating a subject which is free from values, this has given economics a quantitative *bias*.

Unfortunately, many of the most important aspects of the economy, particularly those most directly affecting health and the quality of life, are ones that it is difficult to quantify, and these have therefore tended to be played down within mainstream economics. For example, the enthusiasm and motivation with which people work must influence how productive they are, but how is motivation to be measured? If motivation is measured by output, then how can one distinguish the effects of motivation on output from the effects of other factors? Similarly, many economists believe that the competitiveness of the Japanese economy derives from Japan's cultural and religious traditions. How can these be quantified?

Our argument here is not that such quantification is impossible, but that some factors clearly lend themselves to quantification much more easily and directly than others, and that it is these factors that will gain more prominence in a subject discipline that places so high a value on numbers. In some cases, concepts with very little validity, such as GNP, take on a central significance within economics which they would certainly lack if they could not be quantified.

*Strictly speaking, Y = GNP minus capital depreciation

It is therefore necessary to redress the balance by drawing attention to aspects of the economy that are less easy to express mathematically. Doing so will be seen as value-laden and political, and of course it is. But no more so than existing mainstream economics, for all its 'scientific' pretensions. Those factors that can easily be quantified – like the price of a loaf of bread – are no more real than those that cannot, like its taste, or those somewhere in between, like its nutritional value. The next section looks at the implications of taking the quantitative bias out of economics.

Rethinking economics

Health economics

It might be thought that a subject calling itself health economics would be of great help in addressing the overall health impact of the economy and *vice versa*. Nothing could be further from the truth, as health economists themselves are often the first to admit. Overwhelmingly, they study not the macro-economics of health but the micro-economics of treating illnesses. As McGuire and his colleagues put it:

> That health is not a tradeable thing is a good starting point for the analysis of health care as a commodity. This is not to say that economics cannot contribute to the analysis of consumption or indeed production choices as they affect health. Notable examples of such contributions are the analysis of unemployment as it relates to health and the consideration of health issues in the literature on the economics of pollution. However, *the majority of studies in health economics are in practice concerned with health care economics . . . It will be appreciated then that the text is devoted largely to microeconomic analysis.* (Our italics.)

Mooney, in his *Economics, Medicine and Health Care*, says the real interest of his book and what is central to its discussion is 'the demand and supply of health care rather than health *per se*. But we need to be careful lest the impression be given that the two can be seen as wholly separate'.

Best and Smith give a good example of the approach required in their *The Economic Evaluation of Health Policy: A Macroeconomic Framework*. An example of estimating the impact of health policy on the economy is provided by Cohen's assessment of the economic consequences of producing a non-smoking generation.

New economics

Attempts have been made in recent years to develop an alternative 'new' or 'Green' economics, outside both the dominant neoclassical/Keynesian mainstream and Marxist political economy. Before trying to assess these attempts, it is necessary first to briefly refer to the main contributions.

A central preoccupation has been criticism of economic growth as an objective. To describe this as an 'anti-growth' view is misleading: the new economists argue that the rate of increase in GNP is a very poor indicator of anything, desirable or undesirable. While denying that a high growth rate is necessarily good, they maintain that a low, zero, or negative rate is not necessarily good either. The desirability or undesirability of economic growth at any particular time depends on *exactly what it is that is growing*. New economics is selective: some parts of the economy should grow, others should not, and some should be shut down completely. Criticisms of growth as an aim have taken two forms: writers such as E.J. Mishan in *The Costs of Economic Growth* have attacked GNP as an indicator, while others have argued (e.g. Meadows et al in *The Limits to Growth*) that the pursuit of growth cannot be sustained anyway, because of environmental and resource constraints.

Once growth as an aim is abandoned, a great many other things must follow. The most thorough clearing-out was done by E.F. Schumacher in *Small is Beautiful*. This set out most of the themes that have been worked on since by the new economics. One is criticism of large-scale organisation and advocacy of decentralisation. Here the arguments of Green economists, influenced more by anarchism than by any other political tradition, have coincided with a very widespread reaction against centralisation and bureaucracy, which has taken place right across the political spectrum. Socialists have placed increasing emphasis on local government, community action, and co-operatives; capitalists have rediscovered the virtues of the entrepreneur and tried to promote both the development of new small businesses and entrepreneurial attitudes within large companies ('intrapreneurship').

Closely associated with arguments about organisational scale are arguments about technology. Schumacher made a major contribution to the idea of 'intermediate technology' and to the argument that Third World countries needed to find a different path of economic development from that which would result from copying the West. Again, this concern for small-scale appropriate technology has found parallels in recent thinking on both the Right and the Left. One of the most marked changes in the nature of the Left in western countries over the past twenty years has been the development of a much more critical approach toward science and large-scale technology. Within the business community, recent developments in technology, particularly information technology, have been held out as the basis for more decentralised and flexible forms of organisation, avoiding the overcentralisation for which the Left has attacked big business, and the Right has attacked central planning.

Similarly, there has also been increasing interest among socialists, capitalists and Greens in debate about the future of work. Arguments have been put forward for breaking the connections between work, employment and income, by establishing a guaranteed basic income from government, and at the same time promoting self-employment, both individually and in co-operatives. One important recent discussion of this is *Future Work* by James Robertson.

On the Right, creative thinking has come less from academic economics and more from pragmatic management theorists, increasingly seeing the need to consider the less tangible and quantifiable factors that orthodox economics tends to play down. For example, in *The Art of Japanese Management*, American business consultants Richard Tanner Pascale and Anthony G. Athos conclude: 'the best firms link their purposes and ways of realizing them to *human values* as well as to economic measures like profit and efficiency'. The whole book is about how cultural differences give rise to differences in management styles. There is not a supply and demand diagram anywhere in it: far from building on orthodox positivist economics, business management theory frequently just finds it irrelevant.

Within Britain, the main organisation promoting the development of a 'new economics' – in a Schumacher rather than a management theory sense – is the New Economics Foundation, which has grown from The Other Economic Summit (TOES) conferences. Their book, *The Living Economy* (Ekins) is a collection of papers, mainly from the conferences, providing a useful overview of the various themes now being worked on. More than half the book is about 'The New Economics in Action', looking at various projects for local economic regeneration, proposals for changing taxation and working patterns, and even for reforming the multinationals. Many of the same issues are discussed in *The New Economic Agenda* (Inglis and Kramer), based on a Findhorn Foundation conference, and in James Robertson's *The Sane Alternative* and *Future Wealth*. In the US Hazel Henderson's books, *Creating Alternative Futures* and *The Politics of the Solar Age* have been influential.

The new economics approach contains many strengths that connect it with the new public health. The most obvious is the concern of both for the environment: the economy affects the environment, and the environment affects people's health. On the basis of this connection, it could be possible to begin to develop a new health economics, much wider in its scope than the simple application of profit-and-loss considerations to health care, concerned with how the whole economy affects health and the quality of life.

Both the new economics as a whole, and a new health economics, are likely to generate increasing numbers of proposals for changes in government economic policies and in the way economics operates and is organised. In Chapter 11 we outline some basic proposals along these lines.

It might well be that within the constraints of orthodox economics it would not be possible to 'afford' these policy changes. If that is so, it may be that what will have to be abandoned is the accounting procedures of the orthodox economists, rather than the concern for health and the environment on which our proposals are based. Orthodox economics and orthodox accounting are not direct representations of reality, and of the real constraints which exist, although that is of course what they are often claimed to be. They are neither objective science nor revealed religion. They are simply part of a tradition in the history of ideas with less and less relevance to the real world.

REFERENCES

V. Anderson, *Alternative Economic Indicators* (London, 1991).

G. Best and R. Smith, *The Economic Evaluation of Health Policy: A Macroeconomic Framework*, Birkbeck College, Discussion Paper No. 78 (June 1980).

BBC, *Face the Facts*, Radio 4, 6 October 1988.

BMA, Board of Science and Education, *Deprivation and Ill-Health* (London, BMA, 1987).

D. Cohen, *Economic Consequences of a Non-smoking Generation*, Health Economics Research Unit Discussion Paper No. 06/84 (University of Aberdeen, 1984).

P. Ekins (ed.), *The Living Economy* (London, 1986).

A. Glyn, *The Economic Case Against Pit Closures* (Barnsley, National Union of Mineworkers, 1984).

H. Henderson, *Creating Alternative Futures* (New York, 1978).

H. Henderson, *The Politics of the Solar Age* (New York, 1981).

F. Hirsch, *Social Limits to Growth* (London, 1977).

M. Inglis and S. Kramer (eds.), *The New Economic Agenda* (Forres, Findhorn Press, 1985).

A. McGuire, J. Henderson and G. Mooney, *The Economics of Health Care* (London, 1988), pp. 3-5.

D.H. and D.L. Meadows, J. Randers and W.W. Behrens, *The Limits to Growth* (New York, 1972).

E.J. Mishan, *The Costs of Economic Growth* (Harmondsworth, 1967).

G.H. Mooney, *Economics, Medicine and Health Care* (Brighton, 1986), p. 23.

R.J. Pascale and A.G. Athos, *The Art of Japanese Management* (Harmondsworth, 1981).

L. Robbins, *An Essay on the Nature and Significance of Economic Science* (London, 1932).

J. Robertson, *Future Wealth* (London, 1989).

J. Robertson, *Future Work* (London, 1985).

J. Robertson, *The Sane Alternative* (Ironbridge, 1978).

ECONOMICS AND HOSTILE ENVIRONMENTS

E.F. Schumacher, *Small is Beautiful* (London, 1973).

G.F. Stanlake, *Introductory Economics* (London, 1989).

P. Taylor, *Smoke Ring: The Politics of Tobacco* (London, 1984).

P. Townsend and N. Davidson, *Inequalities in Health – The Black Report* (Harmondsworth, 1982). Re-published by Penguin in 1988 with Whitehead below, originally published in limited numbers by the DHSS in 1980.

T. Valkonen, *Social Inequality in the Face of Death* (Helsinki, Central Statistical Office of Finland, 1987), pp. 201-47.

D. Werner, untitled, *The Lancet*, 29 February 1986.

M. Whitehead, *The Health Divide: Inequalities in Health in the 1980s* (London, Health Education Council, 1987). See also Townsend and Davidson above.

R. Wilkinson, *Class and Health: Research and Longitudinal Data* (London, 1986).

FURTHER READING

P. Deane, *The Evolution of Economic Ideas* (Cambridge, 1978). A history of economics and political economy.

E.F. Schumacher, *Small is Beautiful* (London, 1974). The classic book of 'the new economics': demolishes conventional positivist economics very effectively in the first six chapters.

P. Ekins (ed.), *The Living Economy* (London, 1986). A collection of papers applying the Schumacher approach to a variety of aspects of economics and economic policy.

James Robertson, *Health, Wealth, and the New Economics* (London, The Other Economic Summit, 1985). A pamphlet outlining connections between the new economics and health policy.

A. Glyn, *The Economic Case Against Pit Closures* (Barnsley, National Union of Mineworkers, 1984). An example of alternative accounting, challenging orthodox conceptions of what is and is not 'economic'.

V. Anderson, *Alternative Economic Indicators* (London, 1991). Discusses GNP and other possible ways of measuring economic progress.

M. Jacobs and V. Anderson, *The Green Economy* (London, 1991). Sets out ideas for how a Green economic system could work.

M. Waring, *If Women Counted* (London, 1989). Feminist demolition of GNP accounting.

D. Kemball-Cook, M. Baker and C. Mattingly, *The Green Budget* (London 1991). Green Party economic policy ideas.

M. Jacobs, *Sustainable Development: Greening the Economy* (London, 1990). Fabian Society pamphlet on using economic policy to protect the environment.

CHAPTER 10

Reinventing public health at home and abroad

Several British local councils have set out to promote public health in line with WHO targets. We spotlight Oxford, which reorganised its environmental health department and involved voluntary, statutory and trade union bodies, firms and the people of the city in a public health coalition with democratic control. Popular participation also has a key part in community nursing which follows. The chapter ends with an examination of national goals for health set in Canada, the Nordic countries and elsewhere, indicating that, for public health to be better promoted at local levels, national policies must be developed that will make the healthier choices the easier choices.

Healthy cities

Phil Fryer

Oxford mobilises fresh forces

A growing band of local authorities are taking major initiatives in health promotion. They include Sheffield, Lambeth, Leeds, Manchester, Greenwich and Waltham Forest as well as Oxford, where the involvement began in 1984 and which by 1988 had created a health strategy on which keen interest focused nationally.

The Oxford approach stemmed from a decision by the local Labour Party, dissatisfied with the response of the health authority and another round of cuts and closures, to commit itself to advancing the city's health in its broadest sense. The initiative led, four years on, to a coherent health strategy adopted by the city council and supported by the health authority and voluntary and community groups. Through this venture Oxford is also contributing to WHO's aim to revitalise the public health movement and improve the health of all by the year 2000.

There are two parts to Oxford's 'Healthy City Strategy'. The first is to offset local health inequalities through housing, planning, recreation, environmental health and other local authority responsibilities. The second part is to develop a radical programme of community involvement in a wide range of health factors: food policies, non-smoking, occupational health and recreation, AIDS prevention and cervical cancer checks, health information and research. The evolution of the strategy led to changes and reorganisation in both the city Labour Party and the local authority. First, the health trade unions lobbied the local Labour Party from November 1983 and by May 1984 had extracted a commitment to form a health liaison committee. Second, activists secured the setting-up of a health working party within the city Labour Party; the working party acted and continues to act as a pressure group for public health within the party structure. It published a policy document on health in the city and, in May 1985, set up a health and environmental control committee by merging the traditional environmental health committee with the health liaison committee set up a year earlier. On the agenda of the new body, which set out to take an integrated overview of health matters in the council, were items that ranged from healthy eating and community fitness to radiation monitoring and acid rain, cervical cancer and AIDS. This new agenda for public health proved attractive enough to secure all-party agreement for major initiatives to be taken.

New priorities – new structures

The political base having been secured, the main protagonists of the health lobby sought to equip the environmental health department with a structure suited to the new policies. The new committee required the health promotion and liaison role to be integrated with traditional environmental health. This role began life in the department of planning, estates and architecture. The transfer to environmental health helped to secure a rapid development of health promotion functions on the foundation of traditional work like food inspections, pollution control, occupational health and housing. The health liaison and promotion section is part of the division of commercial and industrial health. It contains a health liaison officer, an AIDS liaison officer, a home safety officer and two part-time community health workers.

New staff with a health promotion role were placed in traditional sections: a community dietician in food hygiene, building on the food inspection work to develop a healthy eating programme for the city; an energy and heating officer in the housing section, to develop a programme to reduce ill-health and deaths associated with inadequate heating; and a community fitness officer in the occupational health section with the task of offering services to employers.

Concomitant with this structural change came a change of ethos and team spirit. Traditional environmental health lived in the shadow of medical practitioners: the new public health strategy partly satisfied the long-frustrated aspirations of environmental health officers to take on new and challenging work. This process was helped by the recruitment of the new officers, who also had experience of community work.

A hundred targets

To consolidate the new approach within the council, a network of health working groups was set up. The formation of a city health working group in July 1985 launched this development. Belonging to the group were representatives of each council department – housing, city engineers and recreation, planning, estates and architecture, environmental health, personnel, city secretaries and solicitors and city treasury, as well as representatives of statutory and voluntary health bodies. Its first major task was to formulate the health strategy that was then adopted as council policy in January 1986. The second, more difficult one was to get each council department to produce health targets in line with the goals of this health strategy. Another group became necessary, the local authority health audit group, and from this emerged one hundred targets, developed by the seven council departments and then vetted and improved by community physicians before they were published. The targets included more smoke-free zones in the city, the completion of an emissions inventory, safe routes to school for children and the extension and improvement of health screening at work.

The planning department took up the challenge of health data and looked at the feasibility of developing a health database for the city. A by-product was the ranking of neighbourhoods in an index of deprivation, using indicators like housing and employment. This ranking directed attention to the social geography of ill-health, which mirrored the social geography of class. The city engineers and recreation department developed a 'safe routes to school' project, safe cycle routes and a community fitness programme. With 250 staff engaged in recreation and leisure centres, a strong foundation for health initiatives was built. A health and recreation group was set up to examine a number of projects. Two fitness testing systems were bought and are now in use in the community; they offer a test, a computer read-out on an exercise programme geared to a person's level of fitness, and health promotion information on diet and smoking. The system was also used as the basis for a health training programme for recreation workers; a community health bus, as part of the fitness testing programme, is to be acquired.

The city council employs 1,300 people and this gave it the opportunity to pioneer a model occupational health policy. Smoke-free zones were established in offices and workplaces, with courses to help people stop smoking as an intended follow-on. The local project on the prevention of heart attacks and strokes was contracted to advise the city on its health screening programme; the idea is to develop the policy and then extend it to trade unions and employers.

Getting the community to help

Publicity among workforces about the aims of the health strategy and the £24,000 'Healthy Oxford 2000 Campaign' was an important spin-off. The '2000 Campaign' helped by pump-priming joint projects; any department or community group falling within twenty-five target areas can use the campaign fund. The campaign was launched in November 1986 in response to the WHO 'Healthy Cities' initiative. The city distributed a newsletter to every household to inform people and encourage consultation of the public. The newsletter concentrated on eight spearhead projects – heating, home safety, ethnic minorities, cervical cancer screening, AIDS prevention, healthy food, community fitness and non-smoking. A sum of £20,000 was earmarked to encourage community participation. This money is being used to engage voluntary organisations in a joint planning exercise around the concerns of the twenty-five target areas. The members of the city's health committee meet with the thirty to forty funded groups to negotiate a health contract, defining how city and voluntary organisations agree to work together over the following year. This system has greatly improved the performance of both the council and the voluntary sector, in focusing on achievable targets. The setting up of a 'cold-line' by Age Concern – aimed at reducing cold-related illnesses – and the financing of a healthy eating guide prepared by the Oxford Vegetarians were two good examples of this approach.

The local authority has a joint programme of neighbourhood health events, organised in conjunction with local schools and community organisations. The programme includes a doorstep 'heart-fit' project – human MOT (basic health check), a fitness test and a health knowledge assessment. Follow-up is two-fold: an offer of smoke-stop, slim and trim and other personal services and, second, social and environmental services in the form of a home safety and home heating visit and a check on take-up of welfare benefits. The integration of personal and environmental health issues is one of the manifest advantages of advancing health promotion in an environmental health department. The latest idea in this regard is to build up a series of self-sufficient modules of health promotion capable of being offered in many contexts either separately or together. Each module is interdisciplinary and involves the voluntary sector. Each can be offered in a health centre or GP practice or in a community setting. Collectively they can be promoted as a local or city-wide health event. The modules are being integrated into the existing programme of city-wide events based around the town hall, the city's open market, its public buildings, the use of stalls, public space, exhibitions and other opportunities for multi-faceted health promotion as they present themselves.

Contracts with employers

Thirteen health contracts with local employers were signed in October 1987, facilitated jointly by the city, the district health authority and the Health Education Authority. Companies signing included Austin Rover, Unipart, Oxford United Football Club, British Telecom, Oxford Polytechnic and Oxford and Swindon Co-operative Society, representing 50,000-60,000 workers in Oxford and its surrounding area. The contracts stipulated that the employers committed themselves to measures to improve workforce health and aid health promotion generally. In a follow-up 'heart-fit' package, the council and the health authority sought to define the employers' commitment. The package included health and fitness testing, health knowledge assessment, workshops and consultancy on eating, smoking, alcohol, exercise and stress, and other key campaign issues.

The first AIDS liaison post

The most contentious, yet most influential, initiative undertaken by Oxford so far has been the appointment of what was the first AIDS liaison officer in Britain. The post is jointly funded with the Oxfordshire Health Authority, but based in the city's environmental health department. The city has developed an AIDS strategy which includes public campaigning, condom promotion and needle exchange. A mobile exhibition is in use and AIDS work is spurred on by an intersectoral strategy encompassing health, housing, social services, community nursing and the voluntary sector.

The appointment of a liaison officer was made in response to a projection of premature deaths from AIDS arrived at as part of a community health profile. When this revealed that within five years the disease could become the major cause of deaths below the age of 65, action on this matter became the most important priority of the health strategy. The demands on the new liaison officer became so great that the city helped to fund, through a health contract, the employment of a development worker for OXAIDS, a voluntary group. Later, the health authority appointed a third worker to prepare primary care and community nursing for patients with HIV-related illness.

The AIDS initiative set a pattern, followed thereafter by parallel projects on food, heating and home safety, and community fitness. The pattern is: joint recognition of a problem by the council and the health authority; formation of joint working group(s); appointment of officer(s); joint setting up and supervision of related projects. It is a process not without its share of conflict, professional jealousy and personality difficulties, but it has proved far more advantageous to all parties than each doing their own thing. Arguments and criticisms are exchanged to the mutual benefit of professionals and the community. Only rarely in three years of the Oxford experience did it prove impossible for one side or the other to overcome perceived professional self-interests in the interest of the greater good.

The expansion of interdisciplinary forums with the health authority led inevitably to the formation of a monthly strategic planning group for healthy city initiatives. The members are the assistant general manager of the health authority, the district medical officer of health, the director of the health unit, the assistant director of nursing services (Oxford area) and the city's environmental health officer and his team. Mutual criticism is encouraged since both sides fear that the cosiness of a 'bilateral corporatism' could erode the cutting edge of health advocacy. The director of public health criticises housing, recreation and planning in the interests of public health and is criticised in turn for defects in screening services, consumer awareness and health promotion services. Criticism, however, generally acts as a spur toward more systematic collaboration on key health issues.

Partnership

The vitality of the new public health approach in Britain centred on local authorities stems from the fact that the initiative was developed outside medical control. It is a municipal and community model, subject to local democratic control. Work with the health authority and especially with public health medicine means, however, that the secular public health model is supplemented and supported by skilled medical and epidemiological input. This secures the benefits of a non-medical and a medical model working in partnership, the key concept. The new class of officers dealing with public health in cities, whether in newly-founded health units or in environmental health departments, meet their medical counterparts as equals.

Oxford has collated its health strategies and presented a compendium of collectively evolved health policy to councillors. Exchanges of information and experience with other people developing (or wishing to develop) the new public health (Allen) have included a two-day course (April 1987) which was developed with the Health Education Council. Apart from countless informal inquiries, news about progress and problems is regularly exchanged at the Local Authority Health Network which was consolidated in 1987. A division of labour has emerged among cities participating in this network. The WHO 'Healthy Cities' initiative has added a welcome spur to the new public health in Britain.

Though it is recognised that the solutions to major public health problems – like structural unemployment, the distribution of wealth and agricultural policy – do not rest, for the most part, in the hands of local government, there is a growing conviction that local authorities can play an effective part in advancing public health in their communities. This role can be further strengthened by their joining forces to influence the national and international agenda for public health.

REFERENCES

Health Education Authority/Oxford City Council, *A Healthy City Strategy* (London, Health Education Authority, 1987).
P.F. Allen, 'Health Promotion: Action Now and in the Future', in Institution of Environmental Health Officers, *Health Promotion: The Challenge for Local Authorities* (London, Institution of Environmental Health Officers, 1988).

Community nursing
Jean Orr

Moves toward partnership

The time would seem to be ripe for community nursing to rediscover its radical roots. This is suggested by the Report of the Community Nursing Review (Cumberlege Report), which stated in 1986 that the starting point for services should be people's needs rather than professional aspirations, and considered that existing services fail to identify many people's needs in a systematic way. The roots of health visiting go back to the 1800s when community-wide action to combat epidemics developed; health visitors had to work not only with individuals but with whole communities, and to seek to improve health by example and persuasion (Dingwall).

Since the 1950s health visitors have moved from geographical patch-working to being part of primary health care teams within general practices. This effectively removed them from any identifiable role as health workers based in local areas. In 1986 two consultative documents appeared that will have profound implications for community nurses if they are implemented. The Cumberlege Report calls for a thorough overhaul of nursing services, and the second report, Project 2000, proposes far-reaching changes in the professional preparation for nursing, midwifery and health visiting.

The Cumberlege Report stresses that primary health care services should enable people to make decisions about their health on the basis of informed choice. They should also involve partnership with and support for carers and all disciplines and statutory and voluntary agencies, and ensure that the planning and evaluation of services involves people in the community as well as health professionals. Rhetoric about participation and client involvement is to be welcomed, but there now needs to be debate about how this might be achieved and the changes in approach that will be necessary. This will be one of the major challenges of nursing education in the next decade and will have to be addressed within the preparation of nurses, midwives and health visitors.

Cumberlege suggests that community nursing should be centred on geographical areas determined by natural community boundaries. These neighbourhoods, with populations of 10,000 to 25,000, would be served by neighbourhood nursing teams incorporating district nurses, school nurses and health visitors. In this way existing lines of demarcation would be broken down, so that for example district nurses could supervise preventive screening programmes for older people. This new approach would be facilitated by providing common core education for community nurses.

The report highlights the criticism, particularly by health visitors, of general practice attachment. While Cumberlege says that primary health care teams that involve the formal attachment of community nurses to general practices are ideally the best way to deliver care, it recognises that properly functioning teams are few and far between. It also recognises that many health visitors are moving to a more community-centred approach not just because of dissatisfaction with the illness-orientation of GP attachment, but because it is recognised that what affects health is located in the community and that resources of the community networks are a vital part of care. It can also be easier to identify at-risk groups within the community and provide group facilities for delivering health promotion.

Rediscovery of radical roots

An increasing number of health visitors are rediscovering their historic roots and becoming involved in community-oriented activities and development (Orr, 1982). A study by Drennan of 130 district health authorities showed that health visitors are involved in a wide range of community initiatives. These fall into eight categories:

(1) Health campaigns.
(2) Health screening schemes.
(3) The formation of, or representation on, special interest or pressure groups. This covered a wide range of groups, e.g. tenants' association, Sickle Cell Society and under-five resource centre.
(4) Provision of health information at local events such as agricultural shows.
(5) Collaborating with other workers to produce information resources.
(6) Involvement in health education in the workplace.
(7) Using local media for discussion of health topics.
(8) Taking part in community development initiatives such as unemployed groups, rape crisis centres, neighbourhood health projects.

The overall conclusion of this study is that although some health visitors are involved in community activities, there are constraints imposed by large caseloads, lack of management support and scarcity of accommodation and funding. It emerges that health visitors are working with a wide range of clients and come under pressure from policy-makers to get more involved with older people. Phillipson and Strang found that this work was very patchy. A series of articles in the *Health Visitor* in 1986 showed some of the diversity of the work.

Progress nonetheless

A number of community nurses are involved in working with women at a community level, and many innovatory schemes are described in *A New Voice for Health*. The women's health movement is a good example of how women have challenged the health care professionals and spearheaded a nationwide movement. In the north-west of England, for example, there is a strong, articulate body of women who have succeeded in setting up women's health classes and self-help groups and have thus been instrumental in changing policy and establishing well women clinics. While these lay and professional women are from diverse backgrounds, they appear united in their demand for health care on their terms (Orr, 1987).

The well women clinics show how lay and professional women have influenced policies and provided a very different service from that of a cytology or family planning clinic. The emphasis is on helping the women identify their own health and social needs by taking a holistic approach. The women are invited to join a range of self-help groups and attend sessions on health problems such as depression.

The well women clinics are examples of the move to partnership and reflect much of the current rhetoric about health care. They are concerned with developing prevention, meeting local articulated needs, involving local communities and forming partnerships, using voluntary and lay helpers, basing their work on a self-help ethos, reaching clients not covered by existing services, bringing together a range of disciplines, and taking a holistic approach to care.

It would seem that community nursing work has to encompass these features if it is to address the health needs of the future. It would also need to promote a public health or environmental perspective within this work.

REFERENCES

A New Voice for Health (National Community Health Resource, London, 1988).

R. Dingwall, 'Collectivism, Regionalism and Feminism. Health Visiting and British Social Policy 1850-1975', *Journal of Social Policy*, 63 (1976).

V. Drennan, 'Developments in Health Visiting', *Health Visitor*, 59, 4 (1986).

Health Visitor, 59, 10 (1986). A series of articles on health visiting and the elderly.

J. Orr, 'Health Visiting in the United Kingdom', in L. Hockey (ed.), *Recent Advances in Nursing: Primary Care* (Edinburgh, 1982).

J. Orr (ed.), *Women's Health in the Community* (Chichester, 1987).

C. Phillipson and P. Strang, *Training and Education for an Ageing Society: New Perspectives for the Health and Social Services* (London, Health Education Council in association with University of Keele, 1986).

Project 2000. A New Preparation for Practice (UKCC, 23 Portland Place, London W1N 3AH, 1986).

Report of the Community Nursing Review. Neighbourhood Nursing – A Focus for Care (The Cumberlege Report) (London, 1986).

FURTHER READING

J. Orr, 'Assessing Individual and Family Health Needs', in J. Orr and K. Luker (eds.), *Health Visiting* (Oxford, 1985). This chapter sets out the background and philosophy of the child development programme and describes the approach taken by health visitors working in this way. There are also examples of the material and cartoons used in this programme.

C. Webb, *Feminist Practice in Women's Health Care* (Chichester, 1986). This book brings together material from nurses and others who are working within a feminist perspective in delivering health care. The book also demonstrates approaches to health care which are non-traditional.

A. While, *Research in Preventive Community Nursing Care* (Chichester, 1986). This book includes a wide range of research-based material covering many aspects of community health and shows the work of nurses with a wide range of client groups.

National and international health goals and healthy public policy

Trevor Hancock

In earlier chapters people's health has been shown to depend on many sectors of society as well as on central and local government and health authorities. Although the new public health places a strong emphasis on participation, there are limits to what a local community can do in the face of nationally or regionally derived unemployment, poverty or other health hazards, including health-damaging policies in different sectors such as agriculture and transport. If we are to reinvent public health at the community level, we need to ensure that national policies and programmes establish frameworks and directions that will enable communities and individuals to exercise more control over their own health and to improve it. That is why national goals for health, national planning for health and public policies that make healthy choices the easy choices must all be developed. And national goals and national planning must be understood to cover areas well beyond the confines of health services; they can help make clear that health is not the concern solely of ministries of health and health sectors, but touches all departments of government and all sections of society. Public policy must be health-conscious in many fields. It cannot (and should not try to) force people to be healthy but it can make it easier for people to make healthy choices. This section examines issues in the two areas of national goal-setting and healthy public policy, with particular reference to North America and the Nordic countries. In conclusion, it looks at some of the problems we face under both headings and at some of the prospects.

Health goals

In 1974 the Canadian Department of National Health and Welfare published *A New Perspective on the Health of Canadians*, more commonly referred to as the Lalonde Report (Health and Welfare Canada). As Milton Terris noted:

> The Lalonde report saw further and more clearly than did the practitioners of public health, bound as they were by the limitations imposed by their daily tasks. The report illuminates the road ahead; it

provides the vision which public health workers need to create what will undoubtedly be a new Golden Age of public health practice.

The Report drew heavily on the work of Professor Thomas McKeown in developing its main thesis that major improvements in health would result not so much from improvements in the health care system and our knowledge of human biology as from improvements in our lifestyle and our environment. The Lalonde Report proposed five strategies, one of which was goal-setting. Curiously, there was little effective implementation of the Report, and in particular no significant action was taken to set goals (Hancock, 1986). In part, this omission was due to Canada's peculiar constitutional arrangement that makes health a provincial responsibility. The federal government has no direct responsibility for health or the provision of health services, except for the military, prisons and on native reservations. What role the federal government does have it has acquired through funding provincial health programmes – although the programmes are still developed and administered by the provinces. It thus proved difficult, if not impossible, for the federal government at that time to develop a set of national health goals and a national health strategy. It was left to the ten provinces to develop health goals and health strategies, and no progress was made. However, two provinces, Quebec and Ontario, subsequently worked on such developments, as will be described later.

The next major step was taken in the US, where two reports in the latter days of the Carter administration established a set of goals and specific objectives for America. Although the federal government, as in Canada, does not have direct jurisdiction, the setting out of these specific targets has provided a model that state and local jurisdictions have then followed.

In the first report, *Healthy People* (US Surgeon General, 1979), health status was reviewed and a broad health goal was established for each age group, usually along the lines of 'overall mortality in this age group will be reduced by x percent by 1990'.* In *Objectives for the Nation* (US Surgeon General, 1980), fifteen priority issues were identified in three broad categories – health promotion, health protection and disease prevention. For each objective an extensive set of specific, measurable and time-limited sub-objectives was established. These were highly detailed, indicating the current situation, the information and resources needed, the activity to be carried out and the outcomes to be attained. A 1985 'mid-course review' by the Office of Disease Prevention and Health Promotion found that while some of the objectives had not been achieved and probably would not be achieved, others had already been achieved and the rest were headed in the

---

*These goals might be better described as objectives, reserving a goal for a 'timeless statement of aspiration' (US Public Health Service, 1979).

right direction. A review of state activities at the same time found that 'many states have made tremendous strides in focusing attention on the health gains that can result from increased emphasis on preventing disease and promoting healthy lifestyles and a healthy environment' (Intergovernmental Health Policy Project).

The one weakness of this generally laudable exercise is that the priorities, and thus the objectives, are very disease-oriented and focused on lifestyles; the entire set of health goals is in effect a set of disease prevention goals. This focus meant that the victims were blamed as usual: that is, society was excused. There is little or no reference to the broad social, economic and political determinants of health that need to be addressed in any comprehensive health strategy. This, of course, reflects in part the level of our knowledge and sophistication about health in the late 1970s, but it also reflects the more individualistic concept of health in the US, as opposed to the more social model of health in much of Europe and Canada.

WHO 'Health for All' targets

These broader issues were addressed in the next significant goals exercise – the establishment by WHO Europe of *Targets for Health For All*. This is, at least nominally, a common European health policy, adopted by the WHO Regional Committee for Europe, consisting of the thirty-two member states. The report identifies four broad areas for improvement:

(1) reducing existing inequities among countries and between groups within countries;
(2) adding life to years by improving people's opportunities to develop and use their health potentials;
(3) adding health to life by increasing the average number of years of life free from major disease and disability;
(4) adding years to life by reducing premature death from diseases and accidents.

This report was a marked improvement on the American report for two major reasons: its emphasis on inequities in health, and the increased attention it paid to 'the political, social, cultural, economic and physical environment that induces individuals, groups and societies to adopt a particular lifestyle' (Asvall, p. 6). The emphasis on inequities in health is particularly important, indeed so important that it was made the first target. The declared aim is to reduce inequities within and between nations by 25 per cent by the year 2000. Whether or not that can be achieved, the mere fact that it is stated as a target is in itself of great value.

The thirty-eight targets identified in the report are accompanied by a set of indicators and a proposed mechanism for evaluation, including regular reporting of progress by each member nation to WHO Europe. This regional WHO initiative has been important because it has induced a number of European nations to revise their own national health policies. In November 1986, five countries had already finished that process, eight others were planning for such new health policies and nine other countries were in the process of making high-level decisions as to whether to develop such a policy. In addition, in two other countries extensive developments of 'Health For All' policy initiatives were taking place at local and provincial levels (Asvall).

The Nordic initiatives

Here we should briefly examine health developments in the Nordic countries. In Finland a new national health policy was approved by parliament in 1985. It emphasises three strategies: promoting healthy ways of life, reducing environmental health risks, and developing health care, particularly primary health care. In Sweden in 1986, parliament approved a report of the National Board of Health on health services in the 1990s. This laid out six clear health policy goals and three areas for action: public policy and prevention, structure of the health care system, and education, training and personnel. Sweden's health policy can be characterised as having moved from hospital policy to health care policy and now to intersectoral health promotion policy (National Board of Health). In Norway a national health strategy for presentation to parliament was nearing completion in late 1986 and the Norwegian Association of Municipalities was involved in developing 'Health For All' materials for its members. A similar process was under way in Denmark (Hancock, 1987).

Contrasts

By contrast with Canada, the Nordic countries have been more successful in establishing national health goals and strategies. In part this is because the national governments have a clear constitutional reponsibility for establishing national policies and standards (with considerable consultation with lower levels of government), while regional and local governments have clear responsibilities for planning and implementing local programmes and services to meet the national objectives. Indeed, one thing common to the Canadian, American and Nordic experience is the lesson that national health goals are meaningless unless they are accepted by local and regional authorities, and unless those same authorities see clearly their own responsibility for actions to attain health goals. Thus the federations of municipalities in both Norway and Denmark were developing plans for the role of municipalities in promoting health and achieving 'Health For All', and the city of Malmö in Sweden had developed an extensive adult education and consultation programme on the theme of 'Health For Malmö'.

Also in contrast to Canada is the recent experience of Australia, another country where the states, rather than a federal government, have jurisdiction over health. A 1986 report from a federally appointed commission (Better Health Commission) indicated the need for a national health strategy incorporating national health goals. A committee jointly appointed by federal and state health ministers developed a set of health goals, which were then approved by the ministers and released at the second International Conference on Healthy Public Policy in Adelaide in 1988 (Health Targets and Implementation Committee). Clearly, federal systems of government are not incompatible with national health goals.

Before concluding this section on health goals, it is fitting to return to Canada. In the absence of a federal or national initiative, the two largest provinces, Quebec and Ontario, have moved to develop health goals. In Quebec, a provincial advisory council proposed a set of health objectives which, while not formally adopted by the government, have been influential within the province (Conseil des Affaires Sociales). A recent commission has also called for a set of general objectives to guide 'a system predicated upon results' (Commission d'Enquête . . .).

In Ontario, a panel established by the Minister of Health proposed a set of seven health goals and thirty-one sub-goals which reviewed and then successfully combined the European and US approaches (a quintessentially Canadian solution!). The seven health goals are:

1. Achieve equity in health opportunities.
2. Enable Ontarians to achieve their health potential.
3. Increase health expectancy of Ontarians.
4. Provide environments which support health.
5. Encourage behaviours which support health.
6. Provide health services which support health.
7. Establish public policies which support health.

(Ontario Panel on Health Goals)

This set of goals incorporates the major elements of the Ottawa Charter for Health Promotion, while the seven sub-goals of goal three incorporate many of the specific objectives of the US model. Furthermore, the panel proposed that detailed objectives and targets should be developed at a local level, in co-operation with the provincial Ministry of Health. Through the Premier's Council on Health Strategy (see below) the government of Ontario promulgated an amended version of these as provincial health goals in 1989. Thus, nearly fifteen years after the Lalonde Report first proposed the idea, health goals were becoming a reality in some parts of Canada and in many other places.

Healthy public policy

'Health For All', as WHO's former director-general Halfdan Mahler has noted, 'is a holistic concept calling for efforts in agriculture, industry, education, housing and communications just as much as in medicine and public health'. An earlier proponent of what came to be known as healthy public policy was Nancy Milio, in her book *Promoting Health Through Public Policy* (1981). She addressed issues of environment, energy, economics and agriculture policy as they affected health, and saw health policy as 'public policy that affects health and not just health services' (p. viii). As she was to state later:

> Policy is, after all, no more nor less than a collective choice on collective lifestyle that sets the terms for individual choices . . . public policy has been and is now more than ever affecting profiles of health and illness, who shall be healthy and how healthy. (Milio, 1986, p.130).

Policy is not simply a matter of collective choice, of course, it is very much a reflection of political power. Whoever holds the reins of power has great influence on our choice of a collective lifestyle, which is why so much of health is about politics.

In 1984 a conference on healthy public policy was held in Toronto to explore the new concepts then being developed (Beyond Health Care). As was stated in the opening remarks at the conference, while public health policy (chiefly concerned with the existing sick care system) accepts the givens of our present socio-cultural system, 'healthy public policy begins by questioning the givens: why do we have to structure our society in such a way as to create ill-health? Is there a way to structure our society so as to create health?' (Hancock, 1985). Healthy public policy has to be seen as part of a wider process of personal, societal and planetary transformation. The implications of this paradigm shift for health includes:

● some shift of attention away from sickness and disease towards positive health . . .

- some shift from outer-directedness to inner-directedness . . .
- some shift away from the currently prevailing perception of the body as a physical machine . . . towards a more holistic perception of health . . .
- a shift in peoples' perception of their responsibilities for their health . . . we shall take more responsibility ourselves . . .
- a growing sense of community and a growing capacity for mutual aid . . .
- increasing numbers of people [involved in] a more active concern for and greater involvement in local community health issues . . .
- people . . . actively involved in campaigning for healthy public policies in every sphere – economic policy, agriculture, transport and so on . . .
- a growing perception of the connections between public policies that are healthy, public policies that are socially just and public policies that are ecologically sustainable [which] will continue to strengthen the links between groups and movements active in these three fields. (Robertson, 1985b)

Healthy public policy was the theme for the 1986 World Health Assembly's technical discussions, under the heading of 'The Role of Intersectoral Cooperation in National Strategies for Health for All' (WHO, 1986). A multisectoral approach has always been one of the key elements of the primary health care strategy; and thus this discussion was attended not only by health ministers, but by over forty ministers and high-level decision makers from other areas important to health, and was co-sponsored by a number of relevant UN agencies (UNEP, Habitat, FAO and UNESCO). In addressing the issue of equity and health, it was noted that:

Relevant health related goals have therefore to be incorporated in the development goals of other sectors, and the health related components of their policies clearly articulated. This is not only essential at the national level, but also must be reflected at the local level. (p. 241)

Three specific areas were addressed at the discussions: agriculture, food and nutrition; education, culture, information and life patterns; and environment, water, sanitation, habitat and industry. Discussions on agricultural policy covered a considerable range of topics, including crop improvements, agricultural extension services, agrarian reforms, investments in agricultural infrastructures, monitoring of food and nutrition, food aid programmes and so on. Healthy public policy is thus a very broad field of concern and action. As was noted in the section on the environment:

> Intersectoral action in health and environment has to be based on the recognition that the ultimate goal of development is improved quality of life and wellbeing for entire national populations. (p. 247)

The great significance that the concept of healthy public policy has come to assume for health promotion and the new public health was evident at the first international conference on health promotion held in Ottawa in November 1986. The *Ottawa Charter for Health Promotion* depicts healthy public policy as the framework for the other four key actions for health promotion (creating supportive environments; strengthening community action; developing personal skills; reorienting health services). The document notes:

> Health promotion goes beyond health care; it puts health on the agenda of policy makers in all sectors and at all levels, directing them to be aware of the health consequences of their decisions and to accept their responsibilities for health.
> Health promotion policy combines diverse but complementary approaches including legislation, fiscal measures, taxation and organisational change. It is coordinated action that leads to health, income and social policies that foster greater equity. Joint action contributes to ensuring safer and healthier goods and services, healthier public services and cleaner, more enjoyable environments. Health promotion policy requires the identification of obstacles to the adoption of healthy public policies in non-health sectors, and ways of removing them. The aim must be to make the healthier choice the easier choice for policy makers as well.

At the same conference, the Canadian federal government released a policy discussion paper – *Achieving Health For All: A Framework for Health Promotion* (Health and Welfare Canada) – which showed the clear influence of the work of the European Region of WHO. Proposing a broad framework for health promotion, the paper identifies the reduction of inequities in health as one of the key challenges and addresses the need to enhance coping skills, strengthen self-care and mutual aid and develop healthy environments. It also identifies three implementation strategies: the fostering of public participation; the strengthening of community health services; and the co-ordination of healthy public policy.

The importance of healthy public policy for the new public health was underlined by the second international conference on health promotion in Adelaide in 1988, where it was the theme of the conference. Healthy public policy was defined as:

> Characterized by an explicit concern for health and equity in all areas of policy and an accountability for health impact. The main aim of healthy public policy is to create a supportive environment to enable people to lead healthy lives. (WHO Europe, 1988)

The conference made clear that we were only just beginning to develop our understanding of healthy public policy and that at that time we had few good examples to follow. (But see Evers, Farrant and Trojan for articles about local healthy public policy.)

However, interesting new initiatives are beginning to appear, including the establishment in Ontario of the Premier's Council on Health Strategy in late 1987. This Council, chaired by the Premier and including six ministers, one of whom is the Minister of Health, and over a dozen senior community and health professional representatives, results from a recognition that society and government as a whole, and not just the Ministry of Health, has to be involved in a provincial strategy to achieve health for all.

In its first two years of work, the Premier's Council has begun to get to grips with the broad issues of health goals and healthy public policy. It has developed a vision of what a healthy Ontario would be like, recommended health goals for the province, identified new strategic directions for the health care system and key areas for healthy public policy (child development, adult development/labour market adjustments and the physical environment). It is now working to develop provincial objectives for each health goal and to recommend specific healthy public policy initiatives. Thus the Council is demonstrating the feasibility of undertaking government and indeed society-wide strategic planning for health.

While there are still no national health goals or mechanisms for developing and co-ordinating healthy public policy nationally in Canada, there are signs that other provinces are beginning to act. Recent reports and activities in several provinces have emphasised the importance of such approaches, while a joint provincial/federal national symposium on health promotion in 1989 began to create a national agenda.

Nor should we forget the significant role that the federal government has been able to play, through its Health Promotion Directorate – and particularly through the health promotion contributions programme – in fostering a wide variety of community-level health promotion initiatives, many of them very lay-oriented, community-based and quite progressive.

Once again we can see through these initiatives the important role at the national level for supporting (and nurturing and protecting) community-based health promotion initiatives. Indeed, the WHO Europe 'Healthy Cities' project (Ashton, et al) and its Canadian counterpart (funded by the federal government) are primarily intended to provide a vehicle for implementing health promotion and healthy public policy at the local level.

Healthy public policy: a Nordic example

In the area of healthy public policy a number of initiatives in the Nordic countries are of interest, as became apparent during a recent study tour undertaken by a group from the Canadian Public Health Association (Hancock, 1987). The Swedish parliament, for example, has adopted a broad health programme which includes requiring health education to establish the link between ill-health and social and environmental conditions, and the establishment of an intersectoral committee at government level to examine intersectoral health issues. However, the experience of Sweden and the other Nordic countries in developing healthy public policy should warn us that it is not an easy task. The difficulties are well-illustrated in relation to food and nutrition policy.

The Nordic countries are broadly agreed on nutrition guidelines, as shown by the publication in 1981 of a set of nutrition recommendations by the permanent Nordic Committee on Food and Nutrition, which has subsequently established a working group on food and nutrition policy. The problem is not the nutrition policy; it arises when attempts are made to integrate this policy with food and agricultural policy. While the first has a clear and well-established scientific basis, food and agricultural policy is not about nutrition but about economics, exports, international markets, profits – in short, politics. Consequently, none of the Nordic countries, despite their best intentions, has really been successful in developing a comprehensive and integrated food and nutrition policy.

Norway has been the most successful and is often pointed to as an example of healthy public policy (Milio, 1981; Ziglio). It has had a joint committee of the ministries of health and agriculture since 1974. However, while government commitment is strong, and a comprehensive food and nutrition policy has been formulated, the commitment of the food and agricultural industries is apparently missing since they are still pushing an unhealthy diet. The implication is that while the impact of the policy on diet has apparently been greater than in Sweden and Denmark, it may not have been greater than that in Canada, where there is no joint policy but where industry appears to have got the message about healthy diets, at least to some extent.

In Denmark, on the other hand, it seems that the industry, through the Danish Agricultural Council, is willing and able to take initiatives. The Danish national nutrition policy, established in 1984, has not involved the Ministry of Agriculture to any great extent, and the ministry still sees itself as playing a traditional role dealing with the economics of agriculture and the export of agricultural products. The industry, though, has begun to see the potential profit in marketing quality, and is keen to play a major role in policy, education and so on.

In Sweden, in spite of fairly close relations between the National Board of Health and the National Food Administration, and in spite of two expert reports (one to the Ministry of Health, one to the Ministry of Agriculture) from committees with similar membership and providing similar recommendations, it has not been possible to agree on a national food policy. As an example of the inadequacy of education alone, knowledge and attitude with respect to diet did change between 1971 and 1978, but behaviour did not (except among the wealthy), probably because at the same time the government had a policy of subsidising foods and the foods they were subsidising were usually those on the educational black list. In short, the message and the incentives were in opposition. Small wonder that behaviour did not change, except for those for whom the subsidies were unimportant. However, there is now more interest in working with firms that are willing to try to educate retailers, caterers and the like. Industry is opposed to nutritional labelling of foods though and has not appeared to be too interested in public education.

It would be fair to conclude that while we may reach broad agreement where science is concerned, we will have much more difficulty in reaching agreement where politics and economics are concerned. On the other hand, while the standard of proof required in science is akin to the criminal law notion of 'beyond any reasonable doubt', the standard for politics is perhaps more akin to the civil law's 'on the balance of probabilities'. Therefore politicians may be willing to make or change policy even when the hard scientific proof is not yet in – something that can cut both ways!

It is clear from these examples that, while inter-ministerial co-operation is important, it is even more important to secure the co-operation, and preferably the active support, of the private sector. Advocates of healthy public policy must find ways in which the private sector can find it in its own interest – as well as in the public interest – to adopt policies that are health-promotive.

Prospects for the future

As should be clear from the example of food and agricultural policy in the Nordic countries, healthy public policy is not easy to implement, even when intentions are good and there is a high level of commitment. There are a number of reasons for this.

1. Much though we may fondly imagine it to be so, health is not the only value in society, nor is it necessarily the most important value. Health must compete with other important values in a democratic society, such as freedom, economic well-being and material prosperity. Where health conflicts (or is seen to conflict) with these values it may lose out. One of the important tasks for the new public health, therefore, must be to identify ways in which health objectives can be made compatible with other important societal values, or to be able to demonstrate very forcefully that where health is in conflict with other values there is a solid reason for giving health priority. We have only to look at the decades-long fight against tobacco to recognise the power of arguments of freedom (in this case the freedom to smoke) and the economic well-being of the tobacco industry and all whose livelihoods are linked to it, in stalling and often defeating effective anti-smoking measures. It was not until the case was expressed in terms of the right of people to be free to breathe smoke-free air and in terms of the economic costs of smoking exceeding the economic benefits, that we began to see a real shift in public opinion and public policy.

2. An important additional point about health as a value needs to be made. Advocates of health need to beware of the dangers of 'healthism'. Not only is health not the only (or even necessarily the highest) value in society; those of us for whom it is the highest value must be cautious of a perhaps natural tendency to believe that we know what is best for society and to seek to impose our health-based values upon society. Healthism, bringing with it a dictatorial approach to life, is the complete anti-thesis of community involvement, participation and empowerment, and must be avoided at all costs (WHO Europe, 1984b).

3. Another problem is where the responsibility for developing and co-ordinating healthy public policy should lie. While at first glance it might seem that it should lie with the Ministry of Health, there are several reasons why this may not be the best location. The first, and most obvious, is that it would be far too threatening for the many other ministries if they saw so much power being vested in a 'rival' ministry. In addition, the Ministry of Health, which in reality is a ministry of sick care, almost certainly would not have the requisite policy and economic expertise for the broad range of issues to be addressed. A third objection may be that the locus should not exist within government, since healthy public policy requires co-ordination and policy development not only in the public sector but also in the private

sector, suggesting a joint initiative. At the very least, the responsibility should probably lie at the level of the Prime Minister's office or the Cabinet office.

4. One of the most important problems is the paucity of research and experience in healthy public policy. Virtually all so-called 'health policy research' is, in reality, sick-care-system-economic-policy research and analysis. There is little attempt to explore the health implications of public policy in a rigorous manner, except for the obvious killers such as tobacco and alcohol. The health implications of economic policy may well be identified, but often only as an observation. Attempts to propose economic policy approaches that are health-promoting have to date been few and far between (Draper et al; Robertson, 1985a; Labonte and Hancock). We will need a substantial commitment of resources to undertake the research and analysis that will be required to provide a solid foundation for healthy public policy.

5. Another danger is that the establishment of health goals and healthy public policy will be seen as a task of national government, and the role of local government will be neglected. While there is a clear need for national-level initiatives, these will be ineffective unless complemented and supported by local initiatives. WHO's 'Healthy Cities' project is an example of a project intended to encourage cities to develop health goals, health plans and healthy public policy and to play their role in achieving health for all (Ashton, Gray and Barnard; WHO, 1990).

Health, sustainability and the Green agenda

The concept of broad health goals is new, and we must consider ourselves to be at the stage of preliminary development and implementation. Yet in the comparatively short period of a decade or so the concept has attained considerable sophistication and a number of nations have developed health goals. Similarly the concept of healthy public policy has gained wide international acceptance in a very short period of time, something like five years. Yet it is doubtful whether the full implications of the concept have been realised by many people, although it presents a significant challenge to our present way of life and the policies and structures that support it.

In particular, one can make a good case for strong links between sustainable development and WHO's 'Health For All'. Indeed, when Gro Harlem Brundtland of the UN's World Commission on Environment and Development, met with the World Health Assembly (WHO's governing body) in 1988, she commented that although there is no specific section of *Our Common Future* about health, '. . . the whole report is about health'.

Subsequently, WHO has recognised the importance of sustainable development for health and has committed itself to supporting the concept, while conferences in at least two countries have begun to explore the links between sustainable development and health (Hancock, 1989; Australian Workshop).

A society where maximisation of health was one of the most important social goals would be a very different society. In my view, it would be a conserver or sustainable society (Hancock, 1980), bearing a close resemblance to the sort of society envisaged by the Greens (Capra and Spretnak; Porritt). The emergence of the Greens as an important political force in many parts of the world reflects the growing concern with values that are more health- and environmentally-based, and a recognition that much in our present society is unhealthy, both for people and for the planet. The new society that is envisaged would be environmentally and economically sustainable in the long term, socially just, communally strong, and personally empowering. Clearly, the new public health must identify with those who share such values and espouse such causes, if we are to have healthy people in healthy communities and nations in a healthy world.

REFERENCES

J. Ashton, P. Gray and K. Barnard, 'Healthy Cities: WHO's New Health Promotion Project', *Health Promotion*, 1, 3 (1986).

J.E. Asvall, *Planning for Health: The European Health for All Targets* (Copenhagen, WHO Regional Office for Europe, 1986). Mimeograph.

Australian Workshop, *A Sustainable, Healthy Future: Achieving Health for All in a Secure Environment* (Melbourne, 1989).

Better Health Commission, *Looking Forward to Better Health* (Canberra, 1986), Vol. I.

'Beyond Health Care [Proceedings]', *Canadian Journal of Public Health*, 76, Supplement 1 (1985).

F. Capra and C. Spretnak, *Green Politics* (New York, 1984).

Commission d'Enquête sur les Services de Santé et les Services Sociaux [English Summary] (Quebec City, 1988).

Conseil des Affaires Sociales, *Objective: A Health Concept in Quebec*, transl. Mercedes Gayk (Ottawa, Canadian Hospital Association, 1986).

P. Draper, G. Best and J. Dennis, 'Health and Wealth', *Royal Society of Health Journal*, 97 (1977).

A. Evers, W. Farrant and A. Trojan (eds.), *Healthy Public Policy at the Local Level* (Frankfurt, 1990).

T. Hancock, 'Beyond Health Care: From Public Health Policy to Healthy Public Policy', *Canadian Journal of Public Health*, 76, Supplement 1 (1985).

T. Hancock, 'The Conserver Society: Prospects for a Healthier Future', *Canadian Family Physician*, 26 (1980).

T. Hancock, 'Healthy Public Policy in the Nordic Countries: Preliminary Report', *Canadian Journal of Public Health*, 78, 1 (1987).

T. Hancock, 'Lalonde and Beyond: Looking Back at "A New Perspective on the Health of Canadians"', *Health Promotion*, 1, 1 (1986).

T. Hancock, *Sustaining Health: Achieving Health for All in a Secure Environment* (Toronto, Faculty of Environmental Studies, York University, 1989).

Health and Welfare Canada, *Achieving Health for All: A Framework for Health Promotion* (Ottawa, 1986).

Health and Welfare Canada, *A New Perspective on the Health of Canadians* (The Lalonde Report) (Ottawa, 1974).

Health Targets and Implementation Committee, *Health for All Australians* (Canberra, 1988).

Intergovernmental Health Policy Project, *A Review of State Activities Related to the Surgeon General's Health Promotion and Disease Prevention Objectives for the Nation* (Washington, D.C., 1985).

R. Labonte and T. Hancock, *Healthy Economic Development: Toward a Health Promoting Economic System* (Ottawa, 1986).

H. Mahler, 'Health 2000: The Meaning of "Health For All"', *World Health Forum*, 2, 1 (1981).

N. Milio, 'Multisectoral Policy and Health Promotion: Where to Begin?', *Health Promotion*, 1, 2 (1986).

N. Milio, *Promoting Health through Public Policy* (Philadelphia, 1981).

National Board of Health and Welfare (Sweden), *HS-90: The Swedish Health Services in the 1990s* (Stockholm, 1985).

Office of Disease Prevention and Health Promotion, *The 1990 Health Objectives for the Nation: Mid-Course Review* (Washington, D.C., 1986).

Ontario Panel on Health Goals, *Health For All Ontario* (Toronto, 1987).

Ottawa Charter for Health Promotion (Ottawa, 1986). Also in *Canadian Journal of Public Health*, 72, 6 (1986).

J. Porritt, *Seeing Green* (Oxford, 1984).

J. Robertson, *Health, Wealth and the New Economics* (London, The Other Economic Summit, 1985a).

J. Robertson, 'Person, Society and Planet: The Changing Context for Health', *Canadian Journal of Public Health*, 76, Supplement 1 (1985b).

'The Role of Intersectoral Cooperation in National Strategies for Health for All: Report from the World Health Assembly', *Health Promotion*, 1, 2 (1986).

M. Terris, 'Newer Perspectives on the Health of Canadians: Beyond the Lalonde Report', *Journal of Public Health Policy*, 5, 3 (1984).

U.S. Public Health Service, *Model Standards for Community Preventive Health Services* (Atlanta, Georgia, Centre for Disease Control, 1979).

U.S. Surgeon General, *Health Promotion/Disease Prevention: Objectives for the Nation* (Washington, D.C., 1980).

U.S. Surgeon General, *Healthy People* (Washington, D.C., 1979).

World Commission on Environment and Development, *Our Common Future* (The Brundtland Report) (New York, WCED, 1987).

WHO, *Health Promotion: A Discussion Document on the Concepts and Principles* (Copenhagen, WHO Regional Office for Europe, 1984b).

WHO, *Healthy Public Policy: The Adelaide Recommendations* (Copenhagen, WHO Regional Office for Europe, 1988).

WHO, *Intersectoral Action for Health* (Geneva, WHO, 1986).

WHO, *Targets for Health For All* (Copenhagen, Regional Office for Europe, 1984a).

WHO, *World Health Organisation Healthy Cities Project: A Project Becomes a Movement* (Copenhagen, 1990).

E. Ziglio, 'The Canadian and Norwegian Approaches to Nutrition Policy as a Health Promotion Strategy', *Health Promotion*, 1, 3 (1986).

Reinventing public health – from watchdogs to broadcasters

Chapter 10 considered different levels at each of which a public health approach is needed; we now look at critically important and specific areas like broadcasting, health promotion and new economics. We start with an examination of the implications for public health of the Conservatives' fourth reorganisation of the NHS. We then take a sceptical look at the prospect of better watchdogs – able to criticise from an independent position – emerging in the wake of the Acheson Report. The next section argues that the NHS, as a health service, must develop robust health promotion services as well as better co-operation with the mass media, especially television (whose potentialities in this field are examined separately). National newspapers – particularly the under-press – are considered from the viewpoint of informing the citizen. In the following section, after a scrutiny of the 'economic' and the 'uneconomic', a case is made for changing socio-economic accounting to cover a significantly wider and more meaningful range of social and economic activity. In conclusion we address problems of greatly improving health and safety in Britain's workplaces.

Fourth time around: NHS reorganisation and public health

Ged Moran

Amid the welter of comment on the reforms in the NHS and Community Care Act, little attention has been paid to the implications for public health. This omission may reflect the fact that the Act itself contains only brief references to public health responsibilities. It could be argued that these issues were addressed directly in the Acheson Report and subsequent circular, whereas the latest legislation is concerned more specifically with the organisation of treatment and care services. Even within this narrow remit, however, the reforms have important public health impacts both in the new structures created and, more fundamentally, in their underlying assumptions.

At both levels it is difficult to envisage the emergence of a strategic public health role within the NHS, or to reconcile the reforms with the key principles of WHO's 'Health For All by the Year 2000' strategy, which many authorities have in recent years adopted as a framework for their public health and health promotion policies.

The government claims that separation from operational management will enable health authorities to ensure that there are effective services for the prevention and control of diseases and the promotion of health. Such a change is not necessarily incompatible with the development of a strong public health role; it has been argued for example that a key factor in the decline of the medical officers of health was precisely that they became bogged down with operational responsibilities to the neglect of strategic and advocacy roles.

It is therefore possible to envisage health authorities, freed in many cases from the responsibility (with its accompanying vested interest) for direct management of major acute sector facilities, focusing more purposefully on the needs assessment, medical audit and health promotion elements of their new role. In these circumstances they will have a direct interest in much more specific data about local health needs, about the efficacy of medical interventions, especially expensive ones, and about the possibilities for alternative health-promoting strategies. They may be able to find creative ways to use the contract specification and purchasing mechanisms to support public health strategies in collaboration with other agencies.

Realistic prospects

However, this optimistic scenario ignores the political reality that the reforms were justified not by public health arguments but by an alleged management crisis in the acute sector. The secretary of state has unequivocally stated that it is in the acute sector that the success or failure of the reforms will be judged, and the spotlight will therefore be on health authorities in their role as purchasers and commissioners of contracts for acute care. This emphasis inevitably leaves the impression that the broader public health roles of health authorities will not be where the action is, either politically or professionally.

Surveys of staff involved in public health work suggest that the problem of securing management time and commitment for this historically marginalised activity has been exacerbated by the clear political priorities of the reform package. There is little encouragement to recruit new skills for public health; instead, the emphasis on financial management skills (and the lack of a clear commitment to fully fund even this recruitment) suggests that few resources will be available for an expanded public health role except perhaps in medical audit and quality control. Nor are the short-term timescales within which political expediency will demand tangible evidence of success (however specious) easily reconciled with the long-term perspectives of effective public health action.

This sense that the public health role is of marginal importance is heightened by the suggestion that mergers might take place between neighbouring District Health Authorities or between District Health Authorities and Family Practitioner Committees. By contrast, attempts to work with the same population (coterminosity with local authorities), a valuable goal for public health planning, is nowhere mentioned.

At a political level too the changes act against the possibility of an enhanced public health role. On the flimsy argument that there is a lack of clarity between the 'management' and 'representative' roles of health authorities, the reforms deal with the problem by abolishing the representative function almost entirely. Whatever the undoubted failings of the previous structure, it is impossible to see how the abolition of local representation (particularly local authority representation) on health authorities will strengthen the emergence of the shared understanding and collaborative working essential for effective public health action.

A financial interest in accidents and illness?

The proposals for NHS Hospital Trusts also show little appreciation of public health considerations. A frequent criticism of existing NHS practice is that it is dominated by major acute hospitals whose contribution to wider public health or health promotion goals is limited. However, the new Hospital Trusts will have even less incentive to undertake such work unless it is specifically written into care contracts, since it will represent both a cost in itself and, if successful, actually reduce patient admissions and attendances and hence hospital income.

National requirements for the Trusts to provide data are also to be kept to a minimum. Once financial data needs have been met, there is unlikely to be room for key public health analyses on issues such as inequalities or race and health – unless health authorities are willing to pay for them. This financial penalty is bound to affect the availability of information for the new Annual Public Health Reports. In addition the move towards contract-based rather than primarily locality-based hospital admissions will complicate some aspects of the collection of relevant information on health authority populations.

Such pessimism about the reforms may seem premature, but these problems are not mere points of detail; rather, they reflect the inherent difficulties of reconciling public health approaches with market-led health care systems. These difficulties can best be highlighted by reference to 'Health For All', since the government has explicitly endorsed the WHO strategy but unlike many authorities is not actively trying to implement it. How does the new structure measure up to the key themes of 'Health For All' such as inter-agency collaboration, reduction of health inequalities, community participation and the reorientation of health care systems towards primary care?

On collaboration, the reorganisation compounds the formidable barriers which already exist. It further fragments responsibility for many aspects of health care provision whilst offering little guidance on the future of joint planning; provision of timely and relevant information will become more difficult; and coterminosity remains elusive. In effect the government has judged collaborative planning procedures to be unacceptable in principle and is offering instead the 'hidden hand' of the market.

A further barrier to collaboration and to public accountability is that large areas of NHS activity are to become shrouded in 'commercial confidentiality'. For example the new Hospital Trusts – mainly large acute hospitals which will be spending the lion's share of the NHS budget in many localities – are required to meet in public just once each year, to present a document called a 'business plan'. Meanwhile, District Health Authorities, shorn of their representative function, will be largely concerned with negotiating and letting contracts, and increasingly with locally-determined wage negotiations. Inevitably they too will be tempted to expand the unhealthy secrecy which already shrouds too much of their business, by claiming in the jargon of the stock-market that information is 'price-sensitive' and hence cannot be openly debated.

Inequalities

On inequalities the current (post-Resource Allocation Working Party) funding mechanism does acknowledge some element of unequal need, although since this remains based on standardised mortality ratios it remains open to criticism. The granting of tax relief on health insurance premiums for elderly patients represents a further erosion of commitment to universal provision, and will underpin the unequal distribution of and access to private health care facilities. Equally, any expansion of marketed services such as screening is unlikely to help those with the poorest health. The complexity of the new structures and the likelihood of increasing geographical concentration of services (displacing costs of access from the providers to the users) will further discriminate against the less articulate and the less affluent.

Nor should the NHS's contribution as an employer to health inequalities be overlooked. Existing occupational health services for its own staff leave a great deal to be desired, and the cost-cutting ethos of the new internal market will provide little incentive to improve these (although the competition for labour caused by demographic change might force some rethinking). However, proposals for pay flexibility have more serious implications. To date these have usually been discussed in terms of large salary increases for prestigious clinicians, or higher rates to attract scarce staff such as computer specialists. But it would be naïve to imagine that the government's objective is to encourage an upward drift in the overall NHS wage bill. Rather, pay flexibility is intended to complete the process begun by competitive tendering in removing the minimal protection of nationally-negotiated pay and conditions from large numbers of low-paid NHS workers. The health consequences for those staff, both during their working lives and in impoverished retirement, hardly need spelling out.

On community participation, the reforms offer a bleak prospect. Effective consultation and participation is a long-term and sometimes expensive process, not easily reconciled with the need to secure and retain short-term contracts. While the new system may offer welcome encouragement to the expansion of individual consultation (e.g. through patient satisfaction surveys), participation at a strategic level is more problematic. Fragmentation, reduced formal representation, greater secrecy and vagueness about consultation procedures will present serious obstacles to voluntary and community groups with limited resources. Although the role of Community Health Councils as public representatives is restated, there is no indication that they will receive either new statutory powers or enhanced funding to enable them to respond effectively to the more complex structures; indeed, where District Health Authorities merge there may well be a reduction in the overall resources available. The number of Community Health Councils has already been reduced in Wales and Scotland.

On primary care, measures such as practice budgets and strengthened Family Health Services Authorities might be presented as a reorientation of care away from the acute sector. However, as opposition from GPs and others makes clear, the proposals are aimed not at strengthening primary care but at tighter spending control, especially in areas which have historically been somewhat epidemic- and demand-led rather than cost-limited. At the same time, the emergence of Hospital Trusts represents a further entrenchment of the power of the acute sector within the NHS.

Parallel reforms such as the linking of payments for vaccination and cervical screening to the achievement of specific levels of take-up are claimed to be a major incentive to strengthen the preventive role of general practice. However, whilst careful re-examination of strategies to encourage take-up is certainly needed, this simplistic market mechanism is not appropriate. Quite apart from its disincentive effects in precisely those areas where achieving high take-up levels is most difficult, it also embodies a narrow vision of the public health potential of primary care, reducing it to a series of technical medical interventions, rather than any engagement with the wider social and economic conditions which shape patients' lives and health chances. Needless to say there are no bonus payments proposed for those GPs who most effectively highlight poor housing, blighted environments, poverty or unemployment where these are local health issues.

The current reorganisation of the NHS is based on two unsubstantiated assumptions: that the NHS is inefficient rather than underfunded, and that private sector mechanisms can be transplanted wholesale to remedy these deficiencies. From this starting-point the legislation imposes major changes with no attempt to identify their implications for other health objectives to which the government is supposedly committed – most notably the pursuit of a coherent 'Health For All' strategy. If the reforms are implemented as planned, no doubt some districts will find ways of clinging on to a public health perspective and developing imaginative initiatives in collaboration with other agencies and local communities. But the possibility of the post-Acheson Report structures contributing to a major renaissance of public health nationally will be gravely and needlessly damaged.

An earlier version of this essay appeared in *The Health Service Journal*.

Better watchdogs

Peter Draper

What will be the long-term effects of the government's embarrassment at the beginning of 1989, not so much about Mrs Edwina Currie, the fallen health minister of Mrs Thatcher's third administration, but about salmonella in poultry, listeriosis in cook-chill dishes and cheese, and spongiform encephalopathy in cattle? Can the ways of strengthening public health recommended in the Acheson Report be expected to rejuvenate medical and other watchdogs? At the national level there is the critically important proposal for a 'small unit' within the health department to 'monitor the health of the people'. The unit is seen as having a

> co-ordinating brief in respect of other Government departments. In particular, it will help maintain consistency of public health policy across Whitehall, for example, when other government departments are considering decisions (eg on food and agricultural policy or on tobacco and alcohol) which might impinge upon health policy. This would require the establishment of a formal means of consultation between departments. (Acheson Report, para 4.8)

Some of the problems of this kind of departmental co-operation were discussed in Chapter 7. However, the Acheson Report's recommendations about liaison with other government departments about public health policy have largely been overtaken by the subsequent White Paper on the environment. While *This Common Inheritance* was widely criticised for being long on words but short on firm proposals, it did commit the government to retaining a ministerial committee to co-ordinate its approach to environmental issues. In addition, a minister in each department would be responsible for its environmental policies. However, although the environment White Paper covered or touched on most of the relevant issues from a health perspective, from air pollution to agriculture and the dumping of toxic wastes, the actions proposed were typically weak, late or vague (Friends of the Earth). Furthermore, the appointment of ministers like John Gummer and Cecil Parkinson as the first environment 'watchdogs' in agriculture and transport respectively did nothing to inspire confidence.

At local and regional levels the Acheson recommendations about public health advocacy and the security of tenure of medical watchdogs are highly relevant. The committee noted that evidence it received demonstrated concern among public health doctors about their

freedom to speak out publicly on health matters affecting the
population of the district . . . We believe that there is currently
considerable misunderstanding of the MOH's supposed role as an
independent advocate for public health . . . We therefore reject the
view . . . that public health doctors, employed in the public sector,
have a duty or a right to advocate or pursue policies which they judge
to be in the public interest independently of any line of accountability.
In the extreme this would place them in a position above Parliament.
(Acheson Report, paras 5.15-5.16)

The point made has a certain plausibility – especially if one forgets what
an outcry there would be if it were made about judges, so widely considered
to be the glory of the British constitution. However, the Royal College of
Physicians and the Faculty of Community Medicine had put on record in
1985 their concept of the role of public health doctors:

. . . their primary responsibility is to their patients and they must be
free to be critical of NHS management policies where their
professional judgement requires this. (Anon.)

Ashton (who wrote the corresponding editorial in the *British Medical
Journal*) put his finger on the crucial point that the Acheson approach
defines the role of an amoral officer in a bureaucracy who dismisses ethical
and professional responsibilities in favour of obedience to employers'
instructions:

The need for a robust defence of public health has never been as
apparent as at the present time. Yet the Report specifically rejects the
view that public health doctors employed in the public sector have a
duty or a right to advocate or pursue policies which they judge to be
in the public interest independently of any line of accountability. Such
a view seems to me contrary to the tradition of medical ethics,
freedom of conscience and the practice of clinical freedom on behalf
of the patient. It seems to assume that government is always benign
and acting in the public health interest. This is clearly not the case.

Ashton also levels criticism at his own specialty:

The report assumes that restoring annual reports will provide
accountability and scope for health advocacy, despite the general

evidence that community physicians have been avoiding contentious
issues and controversy.

There are two other reasons for rejecting the Acheson line on public
comment about important but sensitive issues. First, the report was written
in a period when central government policy had led to extensive damage to
people's health through sharp rises in unemployment and poverty and had
exacerbated already severe housing problems including homelessness, yet
the bark of the public health watchdogs had been inaudible. Indeed, this
was the situation that led to the foundation of the Public Health Alliance
(Smith; Draper and Scott-Samuel).

Second, as we saw in Chapter 7, censorship of politically embarrassing
comments about the NHS and of sensitive public health reports is now
commonplace. Health authorities and their staff have already been sub-
jected to pressure from above to keep quiet about inadequacies in the NHS
to such an extent that Sir Douglas Black, the former president of the Royal
College of Physicians, discussed the 'closed society' in a leading article in the
British Medical Journal. An accompanying article gave twenty examples of
government and health authority actions to silence staff who had been
publicly critical of NHS resources or services (Smith). These included a
change in the contracts of people carrying out research with Department of
Health money, to stop them publishing results without DHSS agreement.
The previous agreement was that the department would be given an
opportunity to comment on reports before they were published. The
pressure on all NHS staff is clearly reflected in the minutes of the North-
Western Regional Health Authority for 11 September 1984, which refers to
a letter received from the DHSS:

> . . . which asked that Health Service Officers should ensure, when
> dealing with members of the Press, that they do not make statements
> *which could be presented as criticisms of Government Ministers*. He
> asked that NHS officers be reminded by Chairmen (of District Health
> Authorities) of the need to be vigilant when making press statements.
> (From minute no. 160, my italics.)

Another case, this time from Smith, was that of the orthopaedic surgeon
who wrote to people on his waiting list to say that financial cuts in the
health authority meant that they could not have their hip replacement
operations. The then Secretary of State for the Environment, Nicholas
Ridley, wrote to the Minister of Health to ask him to 'silence' the surgeon.
'It seems to me intolerable that employees of the Health Service should
openly criticise their health authorities in this kind of way.' Subservient and

health and/or enhance well-being, for example seat-belt laws, tax on cigarettes and alcohol.

Health promotion as described must be based on a number of principles, to avoid the pitfalls of conventional health education. These principles include: reducing stress in the individual, rather than increasing it because of a perceived gap between healthy and actual lifestyle; incorporating community development and participation and strengthening community action; and empowering rather than merely exhorting people to take more control of and responsibility for their health and well-being. Other principles are to attempt to reduce inequalities in health, in place of health education 'by the middle class for the middle class' which widens gaps between social groups; highlighting the importance of process as well as outcome, for example being part of a discussion group; promoting 'holistic' health – a sense of balance and well-being – rather than fear over matters of relative unimportance; and encouraging participation and a sense of belonging for particular groups, such as smokers or HIV-positive people.

Above all the new health promotion must avoid the fundamental flaw of the old health education: it was based on an individualistic approach which 'blamed the victim', making people feel guilty about 'wrong' behaviour, as though poverty, bad housing and other social pressures were non-existent. 'Victim blaming' makes conventional health education both ineffective and inappropriate for many social groups. The new health promotion, on the contrary, starts from the fact that the main causes of ill-health are socially, culturally and economically constructed and, as with unemployment, are often outside the individual's control.

As we have also seen, the Black Report and more recent work (such as Office of Population Censuses and Surveys; Townsend et al; and Whitehead) have documented the enormous inequalities in health between social classes and between different regions of Britain. The WHO policy document *Health For All by the Year 2000* includes the objective of a 25 per cent decrease in such inequalities by the year 2000. Although the British government was a signatory to the WHO policy, inequalities have significantly widened in the past few years. Strategies to combat them must be part of government policy: for any real impact the will of government is crucial. A local programme is no substitute, although it can partially offset the effects of inequalities. It needs collaborative work, local action by groups of health authorities, local authorities and voluntary and community groups to come together to initiate local activities and pool resources. Money and staff must be carefully targeted at the regions, districts, neighbourhoods and groups that most need them. But local health promotion programmes can only skim the surface of deprivation. An effective strategy must involve the redistribution of wealth and power in society.

Health promotion services in the NHS

Despite the inclusion of the prevention of disease and disability as one of the responsibilities of the Secretary of State for Social Services in the 1946 Act which founded the NHS, and despite ample rhetoric in a succession of policy documents from *Prevention and Health: Everybody's Business* (DHSS, 1976) onward, health promotion in the NHS remains a peripheral and low-status activity. It is only within the past few years that some District Health Authorities have even established their own service and units with only one or two staff and minute non-pay budgets still exist. Many districts are far from meeting the DoH's own guideline of one health education officer per 50,000 population (excluding the district post) and 0.7 support staff to each officer; even this level would hardly bring expenditure on health education to 0.5 per cent of the NHS budget.

The total inadequacy of resources is stressed because a very small service cannot be expected to fulfil more than the basic traditional role of providing leaflets, posters and videos to health visitors and a small proportion of other health workers, together with some support to schools. In other words, a badly-resourced service will find it difficult to move beyond reactive work. Without more resources, the long-term development work essential for a coherent health promotion programme will never take deep root in the NHS. Evidence suggests (DHSS, 1987) that the critical mass for a health education service to begin to fulfil its potential is a minimum of five or six staff.

Some of the large services have taken a step toward the new health promotion by focusing away from the individual and onto the community and the institution. For example, the food and smoking policies now implemented in a majority of District Health Authorities have to some extent tackled the wider environment, by increasing the nutritional value of institutional food or introducing no-smoking areas. However, the adverse conditions such as poverty, bad housing and unemployment that are associated with smoking and unhealthy eating are often either not acknowledged, or mentioned but then ignored.

Outside the local health promotion service, a variety of other services are delivered to individuals by health authorities with the purpose of preventing ill-health. The following are among the more important: first, antenatal services, which include a range of screening tests, checks and health advice aimed at ensuring the birth of a healthy baby; second, child health surveillance involving both developmental screening and vaccination and immunisation to support the growth of healthy children; third, screening for cervical cancer and breast cancer which allows detection at an early stage in their development when curative treatment is possible.

To be effective and useful within the framework of the new public health, all these preventive medical services must be based on the following: sensitivity to the social and cultural contexts in which services are delivered; convenience and accessibility; communication with, and responsiveness to, the emotional and information needs of the people receiving the service – usually women; close collaboration between all the health workers involved; the setting of targets for achievement, continuous monitoring, quality control and evaluation; and sound administration and organisation involving users in the planning and monitoring of services.

Separately organised, unfortunately, from health authority services, primary care is increasingly recognised as a valuable setting for health promotion. It can be defined as the network of services provided by a team of health and other workers from a health centre or general practice base to a small identified local population. The fact that 95 per cent of the population will visit their GP at least once over a three-year period provides an unrivalled opportunity for the systematic offering of individually-tailored advice and to learn about the local community health needs and provide a focus for a response to them.

The decentralised base of primary care should be developed to enable more wide-ranging health promotion through participation in a range of information, activity and neighbourhood health groups. The proposals in the Cumberlege Report for neighbourhood nursing could be pushed forward in this direction, as Chapter 10 has indicated. Links with community health councils could be fruitful here: these are the statutory local consumer watchdogs for the health service who try to act as 'patient's friend' and whose potential for health promotion is under-explored.

Family Health Services Authorities, created in 1990, have great potential for the new health promotion. They are not dominated by the management of acute and secondary care services and the practitioners they manage are more closely in touch with community needs.

The 1990 GP contract introduced health promotion into GPs' Terms of Service for the first time and the decision to remunerate GPs' health promotion clinics represents a substantial injection of resources. However, the opportunity of integrating primary care into the wider network of the new health promotion has been completely missed, as the regulations allow only the provision of individual health advice in tightly defined circumstances. It will be a major challenge for the new Family Health Services Authorities to pick up the cause of community-based health promotion and the reduction of inequalities in health.

While there is clearly much room for improvement in the quality of the health education and preventive services described above, it is only with the recognition of *health protection* as an essential area of activity that the health service will move beyond the individualistic 'look after yourself' model into health promotion – into a strategy that enables health-enhancing choices rather than prescribing and moralising about them. Prescribing is sometimes literally the case, as with the 'Give Up Smoking' kit provided for general practitioners to give to their patients, which features a mock prescription with the sound advice written on it.

To become health-promoting, many health authority strategies will have to be reshaped in two fundamental ways. First, rather than paying lip-service to the importance of collaboration by seeking support after policies have been developed, plans should be negotiated from the beginning in equal partnership with local authorities and community groups and a genuinely jointly-planned and resourced strategy produced, on the model of one or two of the best local strategies for mentally handicapped people, for example. Second, plans should focus not on diseases, like the prevention of heart disease or cancer, but on people in groups within their environments, particularly in the workplace and community. The objection will be made with some reason that such a policy is too wide-ranging to be translated into action. Setting priorities within limited resources is, of course, an important part of the purchasing process. Money and staff should be carefully targeted on a geographical basis to the most deprived communities in a region or district. The process of service specifica- tion and negotiation of contracts introduced with the White Paper *Working for Patients* could offer a major opportunity for the rethinking of the role of the NHS in health promotion.

An essential element of the new health promotion is participation and control by people themselves, including the determining of their own health needs and how these might be met. A democratisation and opening up of the NHS is needed to facilitate this dialogue. The 10,000 community health projects and groups estimated to exist are starting to form a community health movement. This is far from united and cohesive, but several forums are trying to draw the initiatives together.

Some of the projects use community development methods, which have been described as potentially the most effective form of health education (Gatherer et al). However, the aim of community development is not so much to find more effective ways to transmit health messages, as to work with groups to help people to change power structures, increase self-confidence and self-esteem and take control over their health.

Nevertheless community development is not a panacea and can be prob- lematic. For example it is not a way to deal with fundamental issues like poverty, nor a means to resolve or suppress social unrest. It should not give people a false sense of what can realistically be changed.

Projects based within institutions (health authorities, local authorities or voluntary agencies) may give rise to conflicts if successful outcomes are seen by power-holders as a threat. With current financial and political constraints, and in a medically-dominated system of health care, it is difficult to see how community projects will be able to have a significant influence on the organisation and operation of the health system, let alone on the more fundamental changes in society that health promotion for all requires.

These comments do not detract from the very real successes of the community health movement, not least in improving the quality of life for a great many people. Much hope and strength will come from the formation of alliances between projects and groups concerned with health, and even more if such alliances extend to trade unions, ecological groups and the labour movement generally. Community development needs much more support from national and local statutory bodies.

Health education and promotion are required at national level to provide leadership, develop materials and initiatives, fund research, disseminate information, co-ordinate the work of other statutory and voluntary bodies, run national campaigns and – most importantly – challenge the policies of the health and other government departments and advocate health-promoting alternatives within the ministries and parliament.

The Health Education Council, between its establishment in 1968 and its dissolution in 1987, attempted to carry out all these roles and succeeded with some, notably support of work in schools, group work skills projects and, to some extent, questioning DHSS and other government departments' policies. As a semi-independent organisation funded by the DHSS, the Council always trod a fairly precarious path, since its financial support was at risk if it was too outspoken in favour of health-promoting policies that might threaten commercial and government vested interests.

The reconstitution of the Health Education Council in 1987 as a special health authority was accomplished suddenly, ostensibly in order to enable the new Health Education Authority to take charge of the new priority of AIDS-related education. Its location within the NHS should enable the Authority to influence regional and local health authorities positively and to co-ordinate national and local activities to a much greater extent. However, the Health Education Authority has lost its status of a semi-independent body, and its direct accountability to the Secretary of State for Health seems to have weakened its ability to press for health-protecting policies outside the NHS. Although the Health Education Authority initially supported a community development approach and the other WHO principles of 'Health For All', in recent years a more traditional model has taken precedence.

Public education

Alwyn Smith has re-emphasised the substantial evidence concerning the importance of education (and associated aspirations) in determining both health and the use of health services. Education has the potential to assist in transforming the social divisions that affect health. It is also essential for an understanding of how different organisations affect the social and economic environment; for self-respect and a sense of self-worth; and for the development of skills and confidence.

Education is often seen as a set of institutions and as embodied in 'experts'. But everyone has an educative role, everyone is an 'expert'. People know a lot about their bodies and their feelings and need to know more, how to keep themselves well and how to heal themselves.

Education in the 1980s largely repressed rather than facilitated the restructuring of society required for 'Health For All'. It was used to create a more competitive and self-interested society. Stuart Hall has outlined some of the features: the restoration of 'discipline' through the classroom, the cutting of nursery education so women have to stay at home, the return of vocational education for some. Health promotion through general education would include rethinking the formal curriculum and other policies and organisation to encourage democracy, parent and student participation and partnership. Personal and public health issues in their widest definition would be a part of this curriculum, including political education, peace studies, ecology, and the encouragement of personal and social skills. Good standards of literacy and numeracy should also be an important part of general education.

Schools and other educational establishments should be opened up for community use: the sharing of facilities and resources should be linked with community involvement in the life and development of the establishment.

Health promotion focusing on the needs of the under-fives and their parents is a priority. Nursery education and child care for all should be available and parent groups supported. Similarly a liberation of adult education is needed – open access, a wide range of opportunities, chances to shape the content of courses, partnership learning.

Education is a vital part of health promotion. It is not only education about and for health – a specific part of the curriculum – but the curriculum itself, how systems of education are organised, who has access to them, who decides what is offered and taught, to whom educators are accountable.

Mass media

Finally, no summary of the new health promotion would be complete without referring to the importance of the mass media which are examined next in this chapter. Both the government and NHS health promotion services buy or negotiate space in the national and local press, on radio and television for advertisements and coverage as part of campaigns to promote healthier lifestyles. Many NHS health promotion services have nurtured good relationships with journalists, who co-operate in the production of feature articles on health issues. Other services produce their own free papers or newsletters for delivery to all households.

The quantity and quality of coverage of medical and health topics such as diet, exercise and screening, have improved considerably in recent years. However, the media remain a relatively untapped and latently very powerful means of informing and promoting public discussion about the impact of social, economic and environmental (as well as lifestyle) issues on health, about tackling inequalities and fostering community participation. Given the penetration and influence of the media in all our daily lives, the building of an alliance with journalists, editors and programme-makers is a priority. The use of the media needs to be planned (unlike some national campaigns in the past) in concert with organisational and social change and local community initiatives to form an integrated strategy for health promotion.

Conclusion

A succession of major reports in the past decade has stressed the vital importance of developing health promotion services in the NHS. All the major political parties have expressed a commitment to it. Yet it remains a peripheral part of the health service. For health promotion to take on the role we have mapped out for it here, substantial resources are needed to develop coherent policies and provide well-staffed services.

While the strengthening of health promotion within local authorities deserves a big welcome (see Chapter 10), the NHS must have a major responsibility. It needs government support to fulfil this role seriously, which may require a shifting of resources from acute services. Without this support a vital component of the new public health will be severely restricted.

REFERENCES

DHSS, *Inequalities in Health, Report of a Research Working Group* (The Black Report) (London, 1980).
DHSS, *Prevention and Health: Everybody's Business. A Reassessment of Public and Personal Health* (London, 1976).
DHSS Task Force, 'Health Promotion in the NHS: A Report on Visits', *Health Trends*, 19 (1987).
A. Gatherer, J. Parfit, E. Porter and M. Vessey, *Is Health Education Effective?* (London, Health Education Council, 1979).
S. Hall, 'Education in Crisis', in M. Lolpe et al (eds.), *Is There Anyone Here from Education?* (London, 1983).

Office of Population Censuses and Surveys, *Registrar General's Decennial Supplement on Occupational Mortality, 1979-83* (London, 1986).

Report of the Community Nursing Review. Neighbourhood Nursing – A Focus for Care (The Cumberlege Report) (London, 1986).

Alwyn Smith, 'Social Factors and Disease: the Medical Perspective', *British Medical Journal*, 294 (1987).

A. Tannahill, 'What is Health Promotion?', *Health Education Journal*, 44 (1985).

P. Townsend et al, *Inequalities in Health in the Northern Region* (Bristol, 1986).

M. Whitehead, *The Health Divide: Inequalities in Health in the 1980s* (London, Health Education Council, 1987).

WHO, *Targets for Health for All* (Copenhagen, WHO Regional Office for Europe, 1985).

FURTHER READING

P. Townsend and N. Davidson, *Inequalities in Health – The Black Report* (Harmondsworth, 1982). The original 1980 DHSS report on 'Inequalities in Health' did not find favour with the government and was not widely distributed. This is the paperback edition, which has a lengthy and valuable introduction, of what has been called the most important critique of the health service and general health standards since the war.

Issues of the Journal *Radical Health Promotion* (Radical Health Promotion Co-operative, c/o Gordon Macdonald, 13 Layton Crescent, Brampton, Cambridgeshire, PE18 8TS). The journal is produced to further debate and provide an expression of alternative radical opinion on health promotion issues. It is intended to stimulate the grassroots development of radical alternatives, and encourage participation and supportive networks of people with common concerns.

WHO, *Targets for Health for All* (Copenhagen, WHO Regional Office for Europe, 1985). The WHO 'Health For All' initiative is important for its status and the recognition that the successful pursuit of its aims will require fundamental changes in most countries. Signatories should be committed to ensuring the prerequisites for health: peace, social justice, wholesome food and safe water, decent housing, education and secure employment.

Better television and radio

Carol Haslam

No one now doubts the influence the mass media can exert on our everyday lives. Of all the media, it is broadcasting – both television and radio – that has become pervasive. For many it is the primary source of information on national and international affairs; it is the major source of entertainment for most people. Broadcasting plays a key role in influencing our ideas, attitudes and understanding of both ourselves and the society in which we live.

It is difficult to analyse the relationship between individual lifestyles and the forces that may have shaped them, but the fact that the media play some role in determining patterns of living is undoubted. We have also seen broadcasting emerge as a major forum for public debate on social, political and economic issues; this 'agenda-setting' role has been much discussed and much studied by media sociologists, who are interested in identifying the ways it influences policy making. Broadcasting has therefore been a source of great hope and great frustration for health promoters and educationalists, who see its great potential in achieving their communication goals, and yet find access to broadcast decision-making either impossible or difficult. The 1990 Broadcasting Act sets a framework for television and radio in the 1990s. It will enforce structural changes in the existing broadcasting organisations and fundamentally change practice. This presents two major challenges to people concerned with health promotion through broadcasting. They are, first, to understand its structures and imperatives, analysing its present state and future trends and, second, to identify ways of intervening in its processes – promoting its good effects on the community's health and attempting to block the negative effects.

Competition for viewers

Broadcasting, like every other activity, does not operate in a social vacuum. It is deeply immersed in the political and economic structures of contemporary Britain and has increasingly felt the impact of 'the market' on its development. Television and radio have been largely protected from full market forces, despite the fact that two of the four national television channels and many local radio services are funded by advertising. This is because, in television at least, there has been public funding through the license fee for the BBC, and an advertising monopoly to safeguard income for ITV and Channel 4. This has enabled a unique form of public service television to flourish, and to spill over, in some respects, into radio services.

Conservative government policies of competition, free market and privatisation threaten this kind of protection in virtually all sectors of the industry. The next few years are likely to see an explosion of new broadcast, cable and satellite services, all competing for viewers, programmes and revenue. The competition for ratings will become a major imperative in programme-making and scheduling decisions.

Programmes on personal health and fitness have always been popular, as have medical films and hospital dramas. More investigative or analytical programmes on the social and political aspects of health care – of which there have so far been many in the current affairs, documentary and education output of all four channels – could become an endangered species, however. BBC1 and ITV have already reduced the number of factual programmes in their schedules and this trend will grow as more entertainment-based services become available by cable and satellite in the

1990s. These programmes will not only be dropped from transmission, but the very valuable post-broadcast role that they have played on hire or sale to formal and informal educational groups will be diminished. The support activities – helplines or free leaflets – that now accompany many 'social action' programmes will also be at risk when broadcasting funds are low.

Another effect of a full-scale battle for viewers' attention is that the notion of a 'balanced' schedule will be abandoned by any channel that relies solely or mainly on advertising revenue. Reduced levels of funding will also prevent major investment in 'quality' entertainment for all but the wealthiest companies. Consequently a big increase can be expected in the amount of imported, low-cost action drama, soaps, situation comedies, movies and music programmes – mostly from the US and Australia – combined with similar home-grown material, plus game shows, chat shows and studio magazine programmes. Currently an over-supply of such American material, together with constraints applied by the broadcasting regulatory bodies, enables programme buyers to reject the more violent or salacious of such series and films and buy only the best quality material. With possibly ten entertainment channels serving Britain and resources spread more thinly, questions of 'taste' and 'quality' would become secondary.

Regulation with a 'light touch'

Britain has developed a formal structure for the regulation of its broadcasting services. The BBC is ultimately controlled by its Board of Governors, who interpret its charter and respond to public and political opinion. The ITV and Independent Radio systems have been regulated by the Independent Broadcasting Authority, whose appointed members oversaw the work of its employed officers in awarding franchises and monitoring performance. The 1990 Broadcasting Act removed regulatory powers of commercial radio from the IBA and introduced a new regulatory body for national, local and community radio stations other than the BBC. The early cable television operators were controlled by the Cable Authority, which saw its responsibility as regulation 'with a light touch' and the fostering of a good commercial climate to encourage the growth of additional privately owned cable companies.

These regulatory bodies have been responsible for ensuring that broadcasting fulfils some public service remit, does not offend public decency, avoids bias or inaccuracy in programmes and, where appropriate, maintains advertising standards. Advocates of the free market regard such regulation as a barrier between the supplier (the television company) and the consumer (the viewer). Conversely, supporters of the concept of public service television argue that broadcasting's informational role would be hard to justify in commercial terms – since such programmes rarely attract as big an audience as pure entertainment – but that the powerful educative potential of television, particularly in reaching people outside formal institutions, should be an obligation imposed on broadcasters by government.

In fact, since the 1990 Broadcasting Act, the IBA and the Cable Authority have been subsumed into the new Independent Television Commission, which will exert a much looser form of regulation on all forms of commercial television whether distributed terrestrially, by satellite or by cable. Although it will award licences it will do so as much on the basis of financial criteria as on factors to do with the quality of the service. It is also likely that when Channel 4 sells its own advertising space it will become more subject to market pressures and lose the distinctive identity of its early years.

The Channel 4 model

In the 1980s Channel 4 provided a model of how a wide range of groups and individuals can contribute to programme making, and how low-cost community stations could serve specific minority interests and needs. To follow this pattern would require a major shift in government policy and the provision of funds by central government, local authorities or charitable foundations. At present the government has made it quite clear that the financial burden of developing the new media should be borne by private enterprise, so the high cost/high risk nature of such projects means that any socially committed and accountable new services are unlikely, to say the least.

On the other hand, the huge increase in new services that will begin to change British broadcasting toward the American model will require local support both in viewing terms and in generating low-cost programme material. This could provide opportunities for community-based groups to establish relationships with local cable operators. Occasionally cable franchises may require some form of community participation, offering a window of opportunity to set up good working relationships between local health activists and local broadcasters – either with a view to supplying relevant material to news programmes, chat shows, or to co-operating on multi-media health promotion campaigns. At present there are few signs of such local initiatives, but technically there is no reason why they should not emerge in the longer term.

'Product promotion' programmes

Another effect of looser forms of regulation for radio and television will be the growth of commercially-funded programmes. The implications for health are indicated by parallel developments in the marketing of foods, drugs, alcohol and related products. The massive growth of the public relations industry has led to the appearance in many programmes of experts paid to represent the interests of particular companies or industries – and not always labelled as such. The consequence could be, as is already seen in America, the rise of a whole breed of new 'programmes' that are really product promotions, attractive as television material because they are cheap.

Fierce competition for advertising revenue will also lead to a relaxation of controls on both the subject and the quality of broadcast commercials. In 1987 the Finnish ombudsman, for example, opposed the transmission of a McDonalds advertisement, for being misleading to children. Both McDonalds and the transnational satellite services that rely on wealthy multinational clients like McDonalds, Pepsi and other snack food manufacturers, put up vehement resistance. A similar battle is being waged over alcohol advertising – banned in most European countries and recently threatened with banning on British television; ITV and Channel 4 stand to lose £100 million a year in revenue from the beer and wine commercials they carry. The pan-European services, even more vulnerable to such restrictions, are trying to force more liberal laws on advertising and sponsorship through the EEC and Council of Europe regulatory frameworks. That could increase the events sponsored by tobacco and alcohol interests throughout Europe and undo the intensive work done by lobby groups over the last decade.

To resist the gradual blurring of distinctions between programme content and commercial messages, viewers and health professionals will need to renew their lobbying of government and broadcasting organisations to ensure that: 1) advertisements are required to give clear and accurate information about products; 2) product promotions, if allowed, are clearly labelled as such; 3) health-damaging products are denied access to television screens and 4) broadcasters' editorial independence is protected from commercial pressures.

Multinational perspective

Like many other sectors, more and more broadcasting operations are developing a multinational perspective, usually in the form of part-ownership, investment, distribution or co-production. Programme series or whole cable services that have proved profitable in other countries are being picked up and explored in relation to their potential for Britain. The American hospital satellite service (which provides specialist information and programmes for doctors and paramedics all over the US) has inspired the BBC to introduce a similar service as a revenue earner for its 'down-time' transmission space. The service, operated by a company that makes films on new drugs for distribution to doctors, found it difficult to establish a viable business, but in the long run multinational pharmaceutical indus-tries will inevitably be interested enough to support such a service finan-cially, possibly through sponsorship. But who would fund other material on primary or preventive health care issues?

There are many lessons to be learned, however, from successful multi-media health campaigns in other countries. Much pioneering work on AIDS done in California and New York has fed into national and local programmes in Britain. Heart disease prevention projects in Finland, Australia and North America have influenced similar campaigns in Eng-land, Scotland and Wales. A number of international conferences have provided an opportunity to learn from other experiences and to exchange written reports on past successes and failures. Anyone embarking on a new project should read these accounts and should keep careful records of their own experience for others' future reference.

Another area of related activity is health education and the growth of audio-visual resources as an aid in school and community education. The availability and funding of such material is determined by the aims and motives of the originator. Many promotional films on health and medical issues are made each year on behalf of the pharmaceutical and food industries. How far are these films helpful in achieving community health objectives and in what ways could health promoters help or hinder their distribution? What other audio-visual and print resources are available for people working in the field, particularly if the volume of such material produced by broadcasters should diminish?

In America the production of audio-visual materials for training and education has become big business. Whether the materials are needed by educational institutions, community centres or workplaces, resources ap-pear to be available to commission or buy them from organisations specialising in educational software. In Britain the education sector, as we hear daily, is short of resources and unlikely to spend much on health promotion materials. However, if ways are not found to combine possible sources of funds and to generate top quality software for use at either local or national level, commercial interests will fulfil that need with other kinds of promotional material.

New networks of collaboration must be established to avoid expensive duplication of effort and to ensure the co-operative use of the scarce funds that may be scattered over many groups but that together could be put to beneficial use. Entrepreneurs of a new kind are emerging – the fundraisers and organisers of resources who can get important 'public service' projects off the ground. Their skills and efforts are already an essential contribution to any community-based activity, and are becoming so in the less commercial areas of the media.

Collaborate with broadcasters

The expensive nature of television and film make it particularly important that resources are used effectively. A good, well-researched and well-supported series will not only have greater impact as a broadcast, but will hold its value 'on the shelf' for some years. Many projects – like healthy city campaigns – are unlikely to have adequate funds to produce their own audio-visual material, so it is worth trying to develop careful collaboration with broadcasters. The Healthy Cities series on Channel 4 in 1988 provided a good example of how a number of different national broadcasters can collaborate in producing a series, each company making one film on its own city and receiving in return broadcast rights on all the other films. At a less ambitious level, the use of local news services is a valuable way of gaining free publicity for community initiatives.

Health professionals can contribute their skills to the broadcast media in three main ways to achieve public health objectives:

1. By establishing contacts – at both national and local levels – with specialist or sympathetic broadcasters. Most reporters and producers draw heavily on their own range of professional contacts, and not all of these will necessarily have been carefully selected: chance meetings, 'old boy networks' or the strategic placing of experts by public relations agencies may well determine whose views are reflected on the air. The best journalists will however take pride in doing thorough research on an issue, identifying key experts and opinion leaders. Making sure that up-to-date policies and achievements are communicated to such programme makers may not always yield immediate results, but long-term relationships should prove worthwhile and 'raise consciousness' among media professionals.

2. By involving the media – local or national as appropriate – from the earliest stages of any health-related campaign. There are many examples of good collaboration, both from this country and from others. It is much easier for the full value of television's pulling power to be harnessed to community or face-to-face activity if both sides plan for this co-ordination from the outset.

3. By developing programme ideas and pitching them to any of the broadcasting companies. Local radio stations are always looking for

programme material, and at national and regional level BBC and ITV will both take 25 per cent of their output from independent producers and Channel 4 about 50 per cent. Sometimes this can be done through local production companies, or the television company can arrange 'marriages'. Only a tiny proportion of such ideas will ever reach the screen, but those that do can influence millions of people.

Many people working in the media are concerned about the current changes in the structure and funding of broadcasting, and they will need to form coalitions with professionals in related areas who see the likely repercussions of such change for their own work. Pooling resources and working together may be the only strategy for preserving good practice in both fields.

REFERENCES

L. Bailey and C. Haslam, 'Action Through the Mass Media' and 'So You Think You Want to Use the Media', in *Coronary Heart Disease Prevention – Plans for Action* (London, 1984).

A. Karpf, *Doctoring the Media: the Reporting of Health Medicine* (London, 1988).

D.S. Leathar et al, *Health and the Media – Second International Conference, Edinburgh* (Oxford, 1985).

N. Milio, *Primary Care and the Public's Health* (New York, 1983). Particularly Chapter 14 – Competing for Public Attention.

N. Milio, *Promoting Health through Public Policy*, 2nd ed. (Ottawa, Canadian Public Health Association, 1986). Particularly Chapter 12 – Determining the Prospects for Health.

C. Robbins, *Health Promotion in North America – Implications for the UK* (London, Health Education Council/King's Fund, 1987). Particularly Chapter 9 – The Role of Broadcast Media in Health Promotion.

FURTHER READING

F.J. Berrigan, *Access: Some Western Models of Community Media* (Paris, UNESCO, 1977). Traces the emergence of 'community media' in western society, specifically, new approaches to broadcasting in North America and Western Europe.

G. Best, P. Draper et al, *Health, the Mass Media and the National Health Service* (London, Unit for the Study of Health Policy, Guy's Hospital, 1977). One of the first analyses of the part played by the mass media in setting the public agenda on health issues.

P.M. Lewis, *Whose Media?* (London, Consumers Association, 1978). A useful background account from a consumer perspective of the changing structure of broadcasting in the 1970s and 1980s.

E.A. Rubinstein and J.D. Brown, *The Media, Social Science and Social Policy for Children* (Norwood, NJ, 1985). This text examines the role of the media in the transfer of research findings to the market place of social policy.

Better national newspapers

Peter Draper

What have newspapers to do with public health? Since Edwina Currie's altercations about salmonella infection in poultry, the role of getting to the truth about infectious hazards and then communicating it is clear. The press, however, has a public health significance – negative as well as positive – that is as wide as the environmental issues we consider in this book. Indeed, the quality and quantity of information people have about their world shapes and constrains their abilities to make some sense of it and thus to live happier and healthier lives. This also applies to people's choices about policies; choosing, for instance, the kinds of road policies that make it much safer for children and older people to get about. If papers contribute nothing – or worse than nothing – to public understanding of how some countries have successfully redesigned their streets in suburbs, for example, the press contributes to a personal policy fog that is every bit as dangerous as a physical fog.

Ask readers of one or more of the serious national newspapers what they think of the tabloid newspapers and two responses predominate, 'I don't know, I never look at them' and 'Oh well, if you are talking about papers like *The Sun, News of the World* and *Sunday Sport*, what do you expect?' This second response can be accompanied by the correct but strictly irrelevant observation that most people get their news and current affairs information from television. If some 'newspapers' contain almost no news, their millions of readers, not least schoolchildren, are scarcely in a position to absorb it from them.

The first step then in considering better newspapers is to resist the notion that whatever they do simply does not matter, but rather to go on to examine how well they investigate, report and discuss matters of clear importance for public health. Almost any day of any week provides one or two suitable topics but here two are chosen. They are of unarguable relevance to people's health: child poverty and the issues involved in Edwina Currie's resignation.

Child poverty in Britain

As we have seen in Chapter 8 and elsewhere, the distribution of poverty is clearly a subject of health as well as more general interest. The subject was certainly seen as newsworthy by the serious papers when the Child Poverty Action Group published *Poverty: The Facts* at the end of 1988. Indeed, in a prominent summary on page 2, *The Times* gave a concise report of the main points under the headline FIFTH OF CHILDREN LIVING IN POVERTY:

> One-fifth of children in Britain are living on or below the 'poverty line', according to a survey by the Child Poverty Action Group. The figures, drawn from government statistics, and disclosed yesterday, show 2,470,000 children living in families on less than half average income in 1985 – the latest figures available. Children at greatest risk were those in families of the unemployed. Those in single-parent families were also more vulnerable. (19 October 1988)

The other two paragraphs of the report informed the reader that the Secretary of State for Social Security (then John Moore) was having meetings with Treasury ministers about child benefit and that he was 'hoping to win an extra £250 million in this year's spending round to avoid freezing the benefit for the second year running'.

The Daily Telegraph (19 October), while reporting the main findings, emphasised the allegations that poverty had increased under Mrs Thatcher's premiership, but ended with an anonymous official from the Department of Social Security pouring unanswered scorn on definitions of poverty used by charities. Furthermore, the extraordinary delays in publishing such official figures as were available – then three years – were also not commented on.

What did the tabloids find space for on this day? Apart from a paragraph in *The Mirror*, not child poverty. MY FEARS FOR OUR CHILDREN trumpeted *The Daily Express* on its front page, with a report that began 'PRINCESS DIANA publicly stressed the importance of mother love yesterday as criticism grew over the Duchess of York's extended trip in Australia away from her baby'.

The Mail had the same lead but left the Duchess of York out of it, announcing DIANA'S CRUSADE FOR OUR CHILDREN. Not so *The Sun*, which used up most of its front page with TWO FACES OF THE ROYALS and the hypothetical question from Princess Bea, REMEMBER ME MUM? While *The Mirror* had a full-length picture of the Princess of Wales on its front page, the main story was about an attack on one of the workers in Childwatch (which investigates child sex abuse), or, as it said in nearly half the page, SEX KID'S SAVIOUR SAVAGED BY THUG.

Apart from the way the tabloids used their front pages, childhood poverty might have got a mention at the expense, for instance, of part of the story of the policeman who was left nearly a million pounds by someone he had befriended. It consumed about half an inside page of *The Sun* and *The Mirror*. A similar amount of space in these same two papers went on the story that *The Mirror* headlined HUSBAND'S SEX ROTA FOR HIS WIFE AND MISTRESS.

Edwina Currie's resignation

Mrs Currie resigned her post as junior health minister on Friday 16 December 1988. Quite why she resigned was a matter of controversy but what was clear even then was that there was a real and far from new problem of salmonella infection in poultry which affected chickens as well as their eggs. How did the Sunday newspapers report Mrs Currie's resignation? *The Sunday Times* was in no doubt that there was an underlying health problem of public interest and its front page headline blared COST OF CURING SALMONELLA CRISIS IS £200M. In addition to the front page story, a whole inside page went on the machinations to get Mrs Currie's resignation and an editorial comment was unequivocal in saying that:

> Although there is a dearth of information about the spread of *Salmonella enteritidis* . . . enough is known to implicate, in Mrs Currie's original words, 'most egg production' . . . It means the infection is thought to be sufficiently widespread for all eggs to be considered suspect.

How did the Sunday tabloids handle the public health issues? *The Sunday Mirror* set a reasonable example with two angles on page 2. The main story was purely speculation about whether Mrs Currie would be reappointed to a ministerial post. The other story was, however, a short factual report about increasing food poisoning in Britain. As would be expected the *News of the World* wasted no space on public health in its early pages which had to be kept for stories such as TRAGIC MARTI COLLAPSED ON STAGE, I CAME FACE TO FACE WITH THE MACHETE GANG and PLEASE SPY ON MY WIFE AND THE FELLA AT NUMBER 8. However, on the leader page, Woodrow Wyatt's columns included a shrewd discussion of whether eggs were safe to eat. It concluded that there was a problem but cook eggs properly and fear not.

In contrast, *The Mail on Sunday* gave half its front page to a 'major nationwide test by The Mail on Sunday [which] has given Britain's eggs the all-clear'. Below the page-wide headline CLEARED, the headlines concluded '. . . and they passed 100 per cent!' Readers who read the report were told that the staff had bought 573 eggs at 106 stores in different parts of the country. The tests had followed procedures laid down by the Ministry of Agriculture and they 'failed to find even a trace of bacteria'. Readers who persisted would have read that:

The tests in no way imply that all Britain's eggs are free of salmonella – but they do prove that the scare started by Mrs Currie two weeks ago is unfounded and her beliefs untrue.

Sunday Sport gave its front page to the headline of an 'exclusive' report, COUPLE STUFF SEX SLAVE IN BOX FOR 7 YEARS. Page 2 had a short report about eighteen people suffering from salmonella poisoning as a result of eating an infected turkey. An environmental health officer was reported as blaming the outbreak on 'not following proper cooking procedures'. No link was made with the problem with chickens, but an even shorter story at the top of the page said that Mrs Currie had been shunned in the House of Commons tea rooms. After pages about BINMAN TURNS INTO DOG, MY GIRL DIED FOR ONLY £500, RED HOT DICK GETS GERE INTO ACTION, JESUS WAS A WOMAN OUTRAGE and GIRL KEPT IN COFFIN AS SEX SLAVE FOR 7 YEARS the editorial page had its publisher sounding off about 'Edwina's sick yolk'. Apparently Mrs Currie should learn to think before she speaks. She could have put the livelihood of thousands of farmers in jeopardy.

Conclusion

If we begin to examine the millions of hectares of newsprint churned out in Britain from the perspective of public health we will begin to take the state of our popular press seriously. We could, for instance, regularly watch informative and yet entertaining TV programmes like Channel 4's Hard News. We could go on to read about how some other countries do so much better and we could examine, for example, the ownership and control of their newspapers, the role of trusts and legislation. We could also listen to organisations such as the Campaign for Press and Broadcasting Freedom which unsurprisingly has a lot of inside knowledge because many of its members are journalists. The start is to acknowledge a difficult but important problem. While schools have a vital task in getting young people to look at the press critically, the awakening of awareness about the seriousness of the situation cannot be left to schools. Ecological and public health problems cannot wait for new generations of critical adults. Furthermore, the political interference of the Thatcher governments in state schools has made many teachers afraid to touch subjects that have such an abundant political content just waiting for bigots and zealots to pounce on and misrepresent.

Britain will develop better popular papers when enough of us recognise that there is a problem and we begin to ask ourselves, for example, why *The Sun* is our most widely read national daily journal. The owner and the editor know of course. How is it that some regional newspapers manage to combine quality with popularity? It is time for some public knowledge, even if we have to commission or do the research ourselves.

The last word can go to Mick Gosling of the Campaign for Press and Broadcasting Freedom:

> Four transnational corporations now control over 80 per cent of the [British] national and local press. Two companies control 70 per cent of national newspaper distribution. Only 50 or so wholesalers are left compared to 500 pre-Wapping. . . . The Sky/BSB merger is a graphic demonstration that de-regulation, market forces by another name, will deliver broadcasting into the same hands . . . This remorseless concentration of ownership is as big a threat to media freedom as direct government interference, narrowing the range of information and opinion available to the public . . . (*The Guardian*, 6 November 1990)

Better economics and better economic policies
Victor Anderson and Peter Draper

Changing accounting

In Chapter 9 we argued that what is 'economic' depends on how the accounting is done. The most important factor determining profit or loss is what gets counted as costs and revenue, as we discussed in relation to whether a coal pit is judged economic. Accounting procedures ought in general to cover as wide a range as possible of the effects of decisions and possible decisions. If they do not do so, decisions will be taken on the basis of partial information. To widen the range of factors taken into account, it is necessary to change accounting procedures and government economic policies in many ways.

The most important of these is the need for a drive to reduce external costs, that is, costs that are imposed on people who are not compensated for them, as when a chemicals firm pollutes a river without suffering a financial penalty. Even without adopting more radical policies, it would be possible within a market enterprise system to make the polluters pay through taxation and fines. Paying for the full cost of pollution would obviously discourage the activities that create it. Similarly, economic activities that create external benefits should attract subsidies to encourage them, which is the theory that has been operated for subsidies for the arts.

Changes in tax and subsidy systems would automatically register new factors in firms' accounting of income and expenditure, and instantly change many activities regarded as uneconomic into economic and *vice versa*. Taxes might be imposed, for instance, on the use of low-priced natural resources in danger of becoming scarce, on all forms of pollution and on the production of low-durability, throw-away goods. Subsidies could be given to firms that minimise the impact of their activities on the environment or positively benefit health. Employers' national insurance contributions, which are a tax penalty on employing people, should be abolished.

Within the public sector, nationalised industries should receive subsidies for environmental and public health purposes and be penalised for activities which damage these. Accounting for the full effects of policies and other decisions in this way would remove simplistic conceptions of what is 'economic'. Argument would focus instead on what would be the appropriate levels of penalty or subsidy for the creation of nuclear waste or the keeping open of a railway station.

Alternative indicators

At the level of national income accounting, there is a clear case for change, as argued in Chapter 9. GNP is highly misleading as an indicator for all except very limited purposes. New indicators of economic success should be introduced, taking account of a wider range of factors than are included in GNP, and supplemented by specific indicators showing the impact of economic activity on natural resources, the environment and health.

Some people suggest that the objective should be to replace GNP as the main indicator of economic progress by a very substantially reformed version of national product, which could be called *Adjusted National Product*. The calculation of Adjusted National Product would start from GNP and then add estimates for the value of production in the informal and household sectors of the economy, and subtract 'defensive expenditures' made necessary by production which has external costs, such as expenditure on environmental protection, repair and cleaning to compensate for damage caused by pollution, costs arising from unhealthy consumption patterns and so on. The concept of Adjusted National Product is discussed in detail by Christian Leipert in the New Economics Foundation's book *The Living Economy* (Ekins, 1986).

Another option is simply to replace GNP as the key indicator of economic progress by social and environmental indicators, such as Infant Mortality Rate and the annual rate of carbon dioxide emissions. Ideally, the political system should become as sensitive to these indicators as the financial system currently is to financial indicators. What the key indicators should be is discussed by Victor Anderson in *Alternative Economic Indicators*.

Institutional changes in economics

Changing economic thinking and policies requires changes in the institutions within which economists work and are educated. Two examples are the structure of government and the A-level and GCSE economics curricula.

At present, the Treasury has the right to monitor, in a powerful and effective way, the implications of activities and policies in other government departments for its own concerns, principally pegging public expenditure. Any policy that involves spending money, which is virtually any policy at all, may come into conflict with the Treasury. There is a need for other departments also to be in a position to monitor central government as a whole and enter into discussion about policies that cause them concern. One of the recommendations of the Acheson Report is for a 'small unit' within the health department to monitor other government departments in relation to health policy (as discussed in relation to watchdogs earlier in this chapter). For public health purposes, priority within economic policy must be to get the Departments of Agriculture, Food and Fisheries and of Trade and Industry to accept that any government assistance to the private sector includes 'environmental and public health strings', conditions applied to subsidies. Public health interests would also be at stake in discussions with the other big-spending ministries that so strongly affect, for instance, unemployment, poverty, housing and transport. This would be a powerful way of developing healthier public policies.

Changes are also necessary in the education system, to give students a much wider understanding of economics than they gain at present, especially at A-level and GCSE. The courses are limited both in the range of viewpoints and concepts they consider – almost entirely mainstream, very rarely anything Green, never anything Marxist – and in their geographical scope. Students are trained to gain some knowledge of the UK economy and of the theoretical nations where 'perfect competition' reigns supreme, but very little importance is attached to the rest of the world. Where the international economy is considered, issues such as trade in commodities and the workings of the IMF are covered in a way which is both naïve and one-sided. Important branches of economics – development economics and the history of economics, for instance – are ignored, while time is filled with trivial aspects of orthodoxy. There is a clear need now to rewrite both the syllabuses and the outdated textbooks that go with them.

Developing a coalition

Building a coalition for new economics and for healthier economic policies can be considered under three headings: mobilising the public health constituency, contacting known critics of conventional economics and contacting potential supporters.

While the recently formed Public Health Alliance may become the home of new economics among health organisations, some other health organisations have members who think in line with new economics and have an excellent track record on public health campaigns which, one way or another, have brought them into conflict with orthodox economic assessments and policies. For instance, as well as obvious organisations like the BMA, the Health Visitors' Association and the Royal College of Nursing, there are many other sympathetic organisations ranging from the Faculty of Public Health Medicine and the Society for Social Medicine to the environmental health officers' organisations, the Colleges of Health and General Practitioners, and the Family Planning Association.

Apart from the small but critically important group of new or Green economists within and around Green organisations like the New Economics Foundation, the Green Party and Friends of the Earth, many other people have developed a good understanding of new economics and the policies that flow from it. Finally, there are many organisations, ranging from those for cyclists and allotment gardeners to journalists and sociologists together with trade unions operating in the NHS, whose members are potential supporters of a coalition for new economics and healthier public policies.

Conclusion

Fritz Schumacher gave *Small is Beautiful* a subtitle: 'A study of economics as if people mattered'. In trying to improve people's health by paying due attention to the economic environment and particularly to the economic assumptions, theories, statistics and estimates that form the quagmire beneath ostensibly 'objective' economic assessments, we could usefully adapt Schumacher's sub-title: 'A study and practice of economics as if people's health and well-being really mattered'.

For References and Further Reading see Chapter 9.

Healthier and safer workplaces

1. *Steve Watkins and John Miller*

Britain and Ireland are the only two countries in Europe that leave the provision of occupational health services to the voluntary decisions of employers. Yet it is in the workplace that health and safety particularly need to be protected; and it is the workplace that is also good for the promotion of healthy ways of living. The Health and Safety Executive (HSE), one of the UK's most important health-promoting agencies, should be given greater executive status than is the case at present. This would overcome the problem of leaving decisions to employers and improve the poor occupational health provision in small workplaces with the help of statutory standards. Occupational health services should include provision not only for a medical and nursing service, but also where necessary for industrial hygiene, safety engineering, ergonomics and industrial psychology. Specialists in these fields should be employed by the HSE and should work for local services on a consultancy basis. Large employers could continue to provide their own services but these should be monitored by a committee of employer and employee representatives and should include a representative from HSE. Small employers could subscribe to a group service provided either on an industry basis by the HSE or on a geographical basis by the local authority or health authority.

Industry has wider health responsibilities than concern for the health and safety of its employees at work. Industry has important influences on the physical and socio-economic environments. Its products and its advertising and pricing policies influence health-relevant patterns. Employment policies often disrupt community networks through rapid job changes and geographical mobility. Authoritarian and hierarchical work organisation feeds the widespread sense of alienation and powerlessness. Each company should be required to account for the health consequences of its activities and these should be audited by a public body. One option would be to give this responsibility to the local authority health unit, which would usefully augment the role of the unit and of the local director of public health in identifying the factors that influence the health of the community and advising upon action. A public health doctor who was a medical adviser within the health promotion department of the health authority and a medical adviser to the health unit of the local authority (through the former, a health adviser to individuals in the community and through the latter, a health auditor of industry) would have an unparalleled opportunity to address the whole range of influences on health. Many companies operate in more than one local authority area and some systems of co-ordination, through designating a lead authority for each company, would be needed.

The ultimate objective should be a system where the health effects of industrial activity are brought into company balance sheets through levies on health-damaging activities and rewards for health-beneficial ones. In industries like chemicals and food, with their special implications for health, the general powers of health audit should be augmented by the power to appoint a director to the board of the company.

2. Jenny Lisle

Turning to the use of the workplace to promote healthy ways of living, the scope is broad. With management support and minimal outlay firms can encourage employees to improve their health and fitness by promoting sound nutrition, encouraging regular exercise and helping staff to achieve a healthy balance of work and leisure activities. The aim should be to create a work environment supportive of positive health practices based on the belief that a healthy organisation requires healthy employees and that urging employees to 'take more responsibility for their health' without providing more opportunities for them to do so, is pointless.

A commitment to health must come from the top, with senior management leading the way to involve the workplace as a whole. Clear policies on health, for example on alcohol consumption and smoking, should be an integral part of a company's strategic plan and a high priority should be given to workplace health promotion as a vital component of an occupational health service.

In 1986 the Health and Safety Commission announced a wide-ranging programme to extend services in the workplace. The programme is an important stage in the commission's developing policy of promoting specialist advice and services available to employees as recommended in the 1984 Gregson Report. When he launched the action programme the chairman of the Health and Safety Commission said: 'We are failing to control adequately illness associated with work and to ensure the best match between people's state of health and their jobs. Nearly half the UK working population has no access to occupational health service'. An American group suggest that the 'key challenge is to fix the place of health promotion programmes in the workplace within the framework of training and human resource development to which enlightened employers increasingly turn to enrich the work experience of employees and to enhance their productivity' (Bezold, Carlson and Peek).

Health promotion has traditionally concentrated on physiological health and few programmes have been presented in terms of psycho-social health or well-being. This artificial division between physical and psychological health is gradually being eroded as the relationship between positive emotional states and improved health becomes clearer. As understanding of stress and its effects increases, in particular of the relationship between stress and productivity, programmes are beginning to extend beyond an emphasis on fitness, diet and exercise to include the whole field of stress management. The workplace environment itself should be pleasant, close supervision and control should be avoided, and working under pressure to deadlines should be minimised whether in executives' offices or on the assembly line. Management should be participative. People should be adequately trained and re-trained – equipped for the work they do and are suited to. Work systems and practices should be regularly reviewed to ensure they are adequate to meet changing needs. Working relationships should be human and personally supportive and should recognise the higher human needs for self-esteem and personal development.

There is increasing evidence from abroad of the positive effect of health promotion programmes on business productivity as well as on curtailing medical costs. It is argued that promotion of health will prove to be the most cost-effective force in health care and that the workplace will become a focus, both for health promotion activities and as a source of information on matters relating to health. The setting for programmes has so far tended to be the large workplace. For smaller workforces they might be run from a community setting or a group occupational health service, one serving an industrial estate, for example.

Occupational medicine as we know it certainly faces a challenge: can it meet the need to redesign existing occupational health provision to rapidly changing work environments? There is a need to develop a dynamic approach to 'total health care management' in the workplace to ensure that a concern for all types of risks and hazards is accompanied by the provision of appropriate medical care and health programmes. Increasing recognition of stress as a major factor in work-related illness and loss of productivity, together with recognition of the employee as the company's most important asset, is bringing about a more positive attitude to health care in the workplace. At present, however, this positiveness is counterbalanced by an emphasis on short-term goals and financial achievement, which leaves no scope for the development and funding of preventive services.

The costs of the negative effects of work on health are enormous and they fall on employees, employers and the community as a whole. The Health and Safety Executive estimated the total costs of occupational accidents and prescribed industrial diseases for 1986-7 at between £1.5 and £2.5 billion (personal communication, 1987). The inclusion of nonprescribed diseases with occupational causes would bring the full costs much higher.

What has happened to cause so many casualties and serious illnesses? Why has there been an unparalleled number of disasters at work? First we need to remember that we are living in an era of great change. The world we have known is undergoing changes of a magnitude which in the past have occurred very infrequently, some authorities suggest only every four hundred years or so. The industrial era is rapidly evolving into a technological era.

The speed with which changes are nowadays occurring has produced a great deal of turbulence and uncertainty that are very apparent in the workplace. Changes of this order, affecting the values, concepts, beliefs and norms of society, have been described by Kuhn in relation to the narrower field of scientific thinking and communication as *paradigm shifts*, fundamental changes in the basic patterns. In the current situation, a new health paradigm is required to fulfil the changing views and needs of society. Already we can see that this will need to be ecological. There is a real opportunity for a different kind of workplace to play an important part in the development of a new approach to health. The old model of reacting to problems when they arise must be superseded by a much more pro-active approach. Preventive strategies for health, showing recognition of the connections between the physical and psychological health of the workforce and recognition of the significance of working conditions, must become part of each company's operating plan. There is also a need for a comprehensive approach to occupational health which would require coordination of strategies across central and local government departments. Occupational health policy should not be drawn up in isolation but should form part of a coherent strategy for achieving WHO's 'Health For All by the Year 2000' (Harvey). Work should be a central public health concern and the workplace a focus for development and implementation of new health policies.

REFERENCES

C. Bezold, R.J. Carlson and J.C. Peek, *The Future Work and Health* (Dover, Mass., 1986).
S. Harvey, *Just an Occupational Hazard? Policies for Health at Work* (London, King's Fund Institute, 1988).
Health and Safety Commission, *Action Programme to Improve Occupational Health Services* (London, 1986).
Thomas Kuhn, *The Structure of Scientific Revolutions* (Chicago, 1970).

FURTHER READING

P. Conrad, 'Worksite Health Promotion', *Social Science & Medicine*, 26, 5 (1988). A special issue containing a collection of eight papers focusing on the social organisation of health promotion in the workplace rather than on specific outcomes. The papers represent first forays into sociological analysis of worksite health promotion.

CHAPTER 12

Prospects for healthy public policy

Peter Draper and Stanley Harrison

Sound public health depends on political creativity and accountability which cannot be achieved without healthy democratic practices. The formation in Britain of Charter 88 is but one manifestation of a widespread discontent with basic democratic procedures – with disproportionate representation in the Commons, with a wholly rigged second Chamber and with no Bill of Citizens' Rights. Will such discontent lead to significant change?

How far will ecological imperatives force major changes in policy which are also positive for people's health? Jonathon Porritt's prophecy in 1984 that 'within the next generation all politicians and all parties will have to become more or less ecological in their outlook' seems to be fulfilling itself faster than he himself expected. The general trend is to 'ecologise' the Left and the Centre and politicise the Greens.

Four basic areas

What chance of a lusty infancy in the next decade has this policy approach to public health that we have been considering? In particular, will Britain and other countries develop healthier public policies? What are the critical issues? These questions are addressed in relation to four basic areas: the impact of party politics; the state of political practice that is deeper than party-political divisions – the state of democracy; global Greening and finally, the prospects of major changes for ecological reasons.

249

Party issues

Perhaps the most direct influence on the climate of political opinion and its relationships to healthy public policy in Britain is the NHS. Were significant numbers of doctors, nurses and other staff to begin to press for health-enhancing rather than health-damaging policies and practices, they could form a powerful pressure group and help the public to see and value the health implications of proposed changes. However, if the main impact of the further reorganisation of the NHS introduced by the Conservative government through the NHS and Community Care Act 1990 is, as many observers believe, a money-oriented approach and then extensive privatisation, most of the attention will focus on selling treatment services rather than on the *health* of the population. Running Sainsbury's well is a question of selling food products profitably, not a nutritional responsibility to keep people well fed.

How the NHS conducts itself as an employer has direct effects on the staff and patients involved and indirect effects as a social influence. Occupational health within the NHS is an old but still disgraceful problem. If the NHS were to set an outstanding example in the health care of its staff it would be in a good position to encourage other organisations to take health and safety issues seriously. At the most basic level, the NHS should pay reasonable salaries and wages. In fact, the low pay of so-called ancillary workers has been a longstanding blot. Moreover, what 'privatisation' means in practice for most ancillary workers is a worsening in their terms and conditions of work such as wage rates and sickness and holiday entitlements. Outrage at what has been happening to those at the bottom of the NHS pile has led, for example, to the resignation of a Cambridge professor from the local health authority. At a management level, changes in the terms and conditions of senior managers, particularly so-called performance-related pay, incentive bonuses (personal and secret), and short (three year) contracts have a detrimental effect on teamwork with NHS staff and with other services.

Will healthy public policy be in each party's manifesto at the next general election? The answer is that the smaller parties like the Greens and the regional parties have already adopted this approach to public health and the Labour party and the more liberally-minded parts of the other parties can be expected to strengthen their health and Green sections. Despite Mrs Thatcher's sporting of Green colours, there is unfortunately no sign of a genuine will among Conservatives to tackle health and safety issues when, as nearly always, they cost money.

We have seen in Chapter 9 in particular that much can be done at town or city level to pass and implement measures of healthy public policy. The Local Authorities Health Network and the Healthy Cities group are acutely aware that what councils can do is very much influenced by central government. As we have seen in relation to environmental health officers, if the control of local government over its finance or its powers in such areas as housing are seriously eroded, as they have been in recent years, the scope for health-oriented action will be gravely limited. The fortunes of local government are one of the items of deeper constitutional issues that are considered next.

Charter 88

Public health cannot be fully developed and safeguarded without real public participation and accountability. Healthy public policy is impossible without healthy democracy. If large and health-damaging institutions can readily escape public scrutiny and accountability, some of these strong institutions will continue to manufacture illness and premature deaths.

But as we have seen in Chapter 7 and contrary to the view propagated through the media by the Establishment, the UK is no longer a country that practices impressive democracy and politics.

Lord Scarman, giving his reasons for supporting the fundamental democratic aims of Charter 88, said: 'It is a bold attempt to tackle the problem of securing the survival of our human and constitutional freedoms amid the complexities of modern British society'. The fact that Charter 88 grew at a speed that surprised even its founders is itself a firm statement that many people judge that democracy in Britain is sick and wish to do something about it.

The focus of Charter 88 is on a constitutional settlement that would, among other reforms, enshrine civil liberties such as the freedom of association in a Bill of Rights; establish freedom of information and open government; create a fair electoral system of proportional representation; convert the upper house into an elected second chamber; and guarantee an equitable distribution of power between local, regional and national government.

Global Greening

A wide range of conservationist interests, at numerous levels of concern, can be regarded as forming the international Green movement. It cuts across the traditional Left-Right political and ideological divisions. At the start it declared itself in principle against politicians and political parties. Jonathon Porritt's *Seeing Green*, with the sub-title *The Politics of Ecology Explained*, published in 1984, challenged the integrity of all other politics, which he described as 'part of the problem' raised by the slide to ecological disaster. By the end of the 1980s, however, all the parties from Left to Right were underwriting, to a greater or lesser extent, the central Green thesis that humankind was collectively moving toward catastrophe. This trend was supported by a popular consensus in favour of measures to avert impending destruction; in less than a decade a minority concern had grown into perhaps one of the widest majority concerns of today, at least in the developed economies whose unrestrained exploitation of non-renewable resources and many kinds of serious pollution contributed most to the 'end game' situation that is looming.

Reverence for Earth

The 'minimum criteria' Porritt stated in *Seeing Green* for being ecology-minded, or Green, included supporting 'a reverence for the Earth and all its creatures', racial harmony and 'a willingness to share the world's wealth among all its peoples' (p. 10). This commitment to redistribution is highly relevant to the many problems of poverty and bad health that we have discussed earlier.

Porritt held that 'the motorway of industrialism inevitably leads to the abyss – hence our decision to get off it and seek an entirely different direction' (p. 43). By industrialism he meant the shared ideology within capitalism and communism aimed at producing 'growth' and recognising no limits to it. Greens were neither Right nor Left but in the centre and were a challenge to 'all politicians to mend their ways' and develop sustainable economies.

Elements of populism in the programme and its eclectic mix of ethical, idealistic and political aims were widely criticised from the Left at the time, while the Right brushed it all off as unduly alarmist and even cranky. That the politics of this emerging force should have been somewhat naïve and lacking inner consistency was predictable in the light of its still rudimentary state of organisation and its broad social base.

But with rapid growth, and recruits joining both from alienated areas of the conventional Right, Left and Centre, and from virgin political territory, Green politics grew up fast. Some advanced aspirations such as international wealth-sharing and racial peace – placarded as Green aims – were condemned by their revolutionary nature to remain utopian unless the Greens entered the field of real politics.

Light and dark Greens

The 'politicising' of Greens, after they had Greened the politicians, is reflected in an analysis of the extent to which Green ideas have penetrated British society written by Porritt jointly with David Winner and published in 1988. *The Coming of the Greens* recorded the separation out of two bands, a light green and a dark green, on the ecology spectrum. Regarding the very wide 'reformist' or light green band, activities

> . . . as diverse as becoming a vegetarian, signing a petition to stop a motorway or living under a plastic sheet outside a cruise missile base in Berkshire are all held to be green. Among a plethora of different aims the most commonplace is simply to improve the quality of life, to be healthier, to save a lovely old building or to protect the countryside. (p. 9)

For most of the reformist Greens the movement is just the same as the environment movement, this analysis finds. 'Dark green' thinking, however, claims to offer a radical, visionary and fundamental challenge to the prevailing economic and political world order.

> At its most ambitious, green politics sees itself as a global life-saver, an urgent response to fast-approaching ecological collapse. It demands a wholly new ethic in which violent, plundering humankind abandons its destructive ways, recognises its dependence on Planet Earth and starts living on a more equal footing with the rest of nature . . . old-style . . . battles between Left and Right [are] diversionary and obsolete. (p. 11)

The claim is, in the words of the West German Greens, 'We are neither Left nor Right – we are in front'. The identification is with progress (of a new kind), no longer with social neutralism. Alongside these 'different' responses to the general danger, there was also evidence of cross-fertilising between the humanist/ethical Green trend and traditional Left reactions. In a cogent critique of the 'Green capitalism' belief that hope can be placed in the so-called 'sunrise industries' like bio-technology, micro-electronics, recycling and pollution control and in the new 'clean' technologies (such as super-conductors, ceramics and fibre-optics) the study accuses its advocates of promoting the idea that

> . . . nothing is structurally wrong with our present industrial way of life, that all we need is a few new fixes and a few filters on the end of industrial discharge pipes. That idea . . . is used to vindicate the argument that industry can go on growing – 'sustainably', whatever that may mean in such a context – presumably until the end of time. Moreover Green Capitalism can give exploitative, destructive, industrial capitalism a veneer of ecological respectability. That makes

it a potent propaganda tool for industrialists anxious to resist deeper change. (p. 150)

Boundaries and coalitions change

Greens, starting off with a Centrist leaning and concept of politics, are proving unable to remain with it. Everywhere they enter the political arena – as they must to figure as opinion-formers, with a programme to be taken seriously – issues arise that divide the 'reformist' sheep from the 'radical' goats, as happened notably to West German and Italian Greens when they competed with Left parties at the polls.

At the same time the Greens humanise and expand the horizons of the transformatory element in social democracy (not the hard Left, but people interested in alliances as a means to construct a coalition, able to check, then overcome, the hard Right). So the general trend is to 'ecologise' the Left and the Centre and politicise the Greens.

Green support flows from a rich and diverse mix of motives. It also comes interwoven with moral and ethical notions, often descended from the distant past, and a medley of religious and cultural traditions. This is the new movement that the political Left has already found impossible to ignore in various countries, will be increasingly influenced by, and must form alliance with, to overcome the ransacking ethos of so much 'private enterprise'.

Locked for nearly two centuries in a unity of opposites with capital, which revolutionised material production and imparted such lightning growth to every social and economic activity, the Left in both its Marxist and social democratic manifestations has assumed that it would take over and use more equally the fruit of this revolution; 'turning round' the state, so to speak, to achieve an 'expropriation of the expropriators' in one version, and to generalise welfare by placing private enterprise and the profit mechanism under curbs according to the other (reformist) version. Labour also shared part of the capitalist and Left assumption that production could be limitlessly expanded; or at least that expansion could continue until the poor had all been fed and clothed, housed and educated, with their future welfare secured.

Rules for one world

People will have to put some valid rules into an acceptable ethical form, make some new ones, and decide whether they want to survive, and how it can be done. TV has brought animal and vegetable species into the living rooms; their beauty, their fragility, their location and function in the food chain in which all living organisms take part, have poignantly entered mainstream consciousness. The tiniest proportion of species has been domesticated or cultivated for human consumption or other productive use. But the knowledge, forgotten during the long march of urbanism, that species do not live apart, 'in the wild', but live with humans in one world, is re-emerging and increasing.

So we see some revival of the alternative ethic to limitless growth ('waste not, want not') which holds that what is taken out of the world should be put back, that the riches are a patrimony that it is wrong to disperse, that no part of it shall be judged useless by human brain or liquidated by human hand. The duty of replenishment, of husbandry, re-enters the world scene as a new moral imperative, fortified by our survival instinct. Human self-conservation and human conservation of species tend to become more closely linked in popular perception. There must be no 'short lists' of species judged worthy to survive, but only in park or reserve. Unknown dangers lurk in such genetic vandalism, as they are widely recognised also to exist in genetic engineering, eugenic 'policing' of the population, and some forms of experimentation with animals. What is involved in these and similar controversies is a moral question, if of a new kind; morality now stretches beyond our rights and duties within human society to a global definition of collective human rights and duties with respect to the total habitat.

Ethical ideas about the right way for the individual to live supply the chief motivation for many Green supporters; they will make progress, perhaps, to the extent that they are nourished by a new social morality embracing the human environment in its wholeness, and by its activation in successful political pressures.

Prospects of socio-economic change for ecological reasons

A sober examination of the prospects of significant ecological and related social and economic change around the globe in the next few years would inevitably be heavily tilted toward pessimism. Apart from anything else, the track records over the last forty years or so are abysmal. While it is true that the childish dismissals of those who were publicly presenting evidence of ecological damage as 'doomsters' fizzled out some years ago in most countries, action is typically far too slow. Similarly, while it is now far from rare (but certainly not common) for people from the rich countries to understand the indefensible trade, banking and development relationships with poor countries – as discussed in Chapter 5 – nothing worthwhile has yet been done on an adequate scale despite the countless deaths, diseases and disabilities caused by economic and ecological vandalism. Would anyone who took civilised values seriously be prepared to enter a court to try to defend such a record?

There are a few reasons for hope. First, there is a remarkable congruence between the measures needed in both rich and poor countries. In the South and the North we need to wake up and respond prudently and energetically to the ecological imperatives. The problems are often very different on the surface, but the basic need for 'Green understanding' is a common one. For instance, the need for ecologically sane methods of agriculture and horticulture is shared and the principles, such as the need for methods of cultivation that at least preserve, if they do not improve, soil fertility, are shared.

Second, Green issues are now widely reported and the basics are understood by anyone of average education who takes even a fleeting interest in current affairs. Further, respectable and 'safe' institutions (like NASA) regularly confirm the reality of sinister changes like the destruction of the ozone layer. Even governments like the British, which has been notorious for lagging, increasingly recognise the reality of problems such as global warming. It is no longer possible for the Establishment to pretend that there is nothing to worry about – and opinion polls regularly confirm the emergence of a substantial Green profile.

Third, an awareness in the North of the exploitation of the South through low commodity prices, high interest rates and other handicaps has probably grown only from rare to occasional but is now politically significant in church and humanist circles as well as among committed Greens and Third World organisations like Oxfam. The shared social morality is crucial, it makes possible the shared policy aims of people operating from very different foundations of belief.

Fourth, the old economics is breaking down and North and South have a common interest in developing an economics of the kind discussed in Chapters 9 and 11 that is relevant to today and tomorrow and that actually helps us begin to cope with important factors that are difficult to measure reliably and easily, particularly an assessment of social progress that is meaningful and Green-sensitive, unlike GNP or GDP. Further, North and South also have many people who have a common interest in finding ways of analysing basic human needs like food and shelter and silencing once and for all the exponents of the shoddy 'trickle down' theory that excuses so much economic and social irresponsibility.

A new economics also needs to acknowledge that it is far from value-free. And the value content needs to be explicit – and civilised. In rich and poor countries there are millions of disadvantaged people – many at the bottom of the socio-economic divide, which is also the health divide. In rich and poor countries alike we have to awaken our social consciences and refuse to accept starvation, homelessness, involuntary and impoverished unemployment, land sterilisation and all the other results of greed, ignorance, fear and ill-shared power.

Fifth, Mikhail Gorbachev's breaking of the East-West industrial-military logjam increases the possibilities of reasonable international behaviour and has already reduced the risks of either accidental or deliberate nuclear war.

Last, the reader will have noticed that discussions of values, of ethics, of morality, of non-fanatical religion come up throughout this book. This was not planned, though when it began to appear it was welcomed. It is as though current generations are growing out of some kind of spuriously objective scientism, while respecting genuine scientific endeavours, and are emerging from the anaesthesia of mainstream economics and from the claustrophobia of sectarian, party-political bickering and evasion of basic issues while the planetary clock ticks away.

Seeing the interconnectedness of things, trying to develop healthy public policies in unhealthy, myopic countries, may not damage our health, but it can tax the isolated individual. Battling for the new public health can seem like taking on the world. Where do responsibilities end? What can one person do that is worthwhile? One thing that is widely shared in the Green movement is an awareness of Green and health-promoting networks and the need to think globally but act locally. Each of us can make some kind of contribution to healthier ways of thinking and acting – even if it is only through talking with our friends. And each of us can draw strength from Green and healthy networks, from what others have already done and are now doing.

The former WHO director-general, Halfdan Mahler, insists that 'Health For All' is a movement *of* the people as well as *for* the people. Here is the salutary reminder he included in his opening address to the Second International Conference of Health Promotion (1988) in Adelaide, Australia:

Many of the early pioneers were also social reformers, pioneers in the organisation of labour, of education, housing and sanitation. Much of this link has been lost in the development of public health. Social medicine and social policy have taken separate roads. Recent textbooks on public health or epidemiology frighten me by showing how much public health has lost its original link to social justice, social change and social reform and how it has opted for behavioural victim-blaming instead.

In relation to health and to Dr Mahler's broader environment that rightly includes socio-economic aspects, a recent WHO initiative has produced a charter on environment and health adopted by the environment and health ministries of twenty-nine European countries (WHO). The challenge is to turn these useful statements into reality and to develop a more strongly global perspective in relation to resources, pollution and trade.

REFERENCES

H. Mahler, Opening address to the Second International Conference of Health Promotion, Adelaide, 1988. Available from WHO Regional Office for Europe, (Health Promotion), 8 Scherfigsvej, Copenhagen, Denmark.

J. Porritt, *Seeing Green: The Politics of Ecology Explained* (Oxford, 1984).

J. Porritt and D. Winner, *The Coming of the Greens* (London, 1988).

Lord Scarman, 'Why I signed the Charter', *The Observer*, 22 January 1989.

WHO, *Environment and Health: The European Charter and Commentary* (Copenhagen, WHO Regional Office for Europe, 1990).